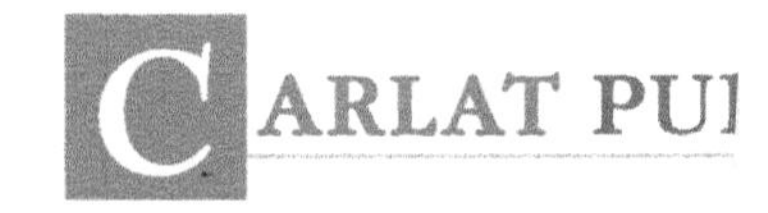

Medication Fact Book *for* Psychiatric Practice

FOURTH EDITION

Talia Puzantian, PharmD, BCPP
Associate Professor, Keck Graduate Institute School of Pharmacy, Claremont, CA

Daniel J. Carlat, MD
Publisher and Editor-in-Chief, The Carlat Psychiatry Report
Associate Clinical Professor, Tufts University School of Medicine, Boston, MA

Published by Carlat Publishing, LLC
PO Box 626, Newburyport, MA 01950

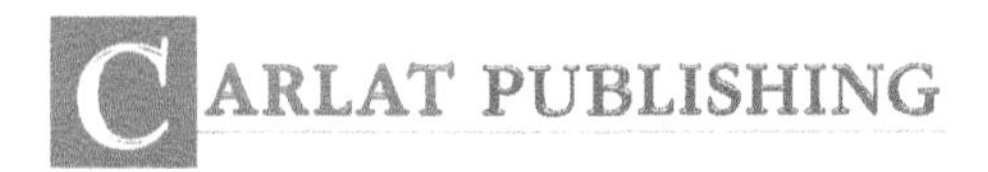

Medication Fact Book

For Psychiatric Practice

FOURTH EDITION

Published by Carlat Publishing, LLC
PO Box 626, Newburyport, MA 01950

Publisher and Editor-in-Chief: Daniel J. Carlat, MD

Deputy Editor: Talia Puzantian, PharmD, BCPP
Executive Editor: Janice Jutras

This CME/CE activity is intended for psychiatrists, psychiatric nurses, psychologists, and other health care professionals with an interest in mental health. The Carlat CME Institute is accredited by the Accreditation Council for Continuing Medical Education to provide continuing medical education for physicians. Carlat CME Institute is approved by the American Psychological Association to sponsor continuing education for psychologists. Carlat CME Institute maintains responsibility for this program and its content. Carlat CME Institute designates this enduring material educational activity for a maximum of twelve (12) AMA PRA Category 1 Credits™ or 12 CE for psychologists. Physicians or psychologists should claim credit commensurate only with the extent of their participation in the activity. The American Board of Psychiatry and Neurology has reviewed the *Medication Fact Book for Psychiatric Practice* and has approved this program as part of a comprehensive Self-Assessment and CME Program, which is mandated by ABMS as a necessary component of maintenance of certification. CME quizzes must be taken online at www.thecarlatreport.com or http://thecarlatcmeinstitute.com/self-assessment (for ABPN SA course subscribers).

To order, visit www.thecarlatreport.com
or call (866) 348-9279

2 3 4 5 6 7 8 9 10

ISBN #: 978-0-9975106-6-9

PRINTED IN THE UNITED STATES OF AMERICA

Table of Contents

LIST OF TABLES

Introduction

HOW TO USE THIS BOOK

Medication information is presented in two ways in this book.

Medication fact sheets: In-depth prescribing information for select medications. There are 115 medication fact sheets in this book. These don't cover all psychiatric medications, but we have included most of the commonly prescribed and newer medications.

Quick-scan medication tables: These are most often located at the beginning of each therapeutic category and list the very basics: generic and brand names, strengths available, starting doses, and target doses. These tables contain most of the commonly prescribed psychiatric medications.

CHANGES AND ADDITIONS TO THE FOURTH EDITION

Medication fact sheets have been updated to reflect availability of newer strengths and formulations, as well as generics. New clinical data have been incorporated into the previous edition's fact sheets. Many categories of medications have been expanded to include a larger number of medications: 14 new fact sheets and 2 additional tables are included in this edition. Side effect management fact sheets have also been added, covering the 16 most common side effects your patients may experience. These detailed fact sheets include characteristics of the side effects, the medications that may contribute to them, mechanism, general management as well as medication management, clinical pearls, and fun facts.

CATEGORIES OF MEDICATIONS

We did our best to categorize medications rationally. However, in some cases a medication can fall into more than one category. In such cases, we categorized the medication with the types of disorders for which it is most often used. If you're having trouble finding a medication in a particular section, look in the index to find its page number.

MORE ON THE MEDICATION FACT SHEETS

The goal of these fact sheets is to provide need-to-know information that can be easily and quickly absorbed during a busy day of seeing patients. Our main criterion is that all the information should fit on a single page. Please refer to the *PDR (Physicians' Desk Reference)* when you need more in-depth information.

For the most part, each fact sheet contains the following information:

- Both the brand and generic names.
- **A [G] or (G) denotes generic availability.**
- FDA-approved indications.
- Off-label uses. We list the more common off-label uses, based on both the medical literature and our own clinical experience. Just because we list a potential use does not imply that we endorse a medication as being particularly effective for that use. We are simply alerting you to the fact that there is some evidence for efficacy.
- Dosage forms, along with available strengths.
- Dosage guidance. We provide recommendations on how to dose medications; these are derived from a variety of sources, including package inserts, clinical trials, and common clinical practice. In other words, don't be surprised when our dosing instructions are at odds with what you find in the *PDR*.
- Lab monitoring recommendations. We include the usual routine monitoring measures for each medication. Of course, you may need to think beyond the "routine" if the clinical picture warrants it.
- Cost information. Pricing information for a 1-month supply of a common dosing regimen was obtained from the website GoodRx (https://www.goodrx.com), accessed in July 2017. These are the prices a patient would have to pay if he or she had no insurance. Because of wide variations in price depending on the pharmacy, in this edition of the *Medication Fact Book* we list price categories rather than the price in dollars. The categories are:
  - $: Inexpensive: <$50/month
  - $$: Moderate: $50–$100/month
  - $$$: Expensive: $100–$200/month
  - $$$$: Very expensive: $200–$500/month
  - $$$$$: Extremely expensive: >$500/month

This begs the question, what should you do with knowledge of retail pricing? After all, most patients have some type of insurance and are therefore not going to pay retail price, but rather a co-pay. Since there's no clear source for accurately predicting a co-pay, you can use the retail price as a clue. Meds that are very inexpensive will likely require no co-pay, while the most expensive drugs will either require a very expensive co-pay, or, more likely, will not be covered at all without an onerous pre-authorization process.

- Side effects information. We break down side effects into "most common" vs "rare but serious" side effects. We generally define "most common" side effects as those occurring in at least 5% of patients in clinical trials, and which were at least double the rate of the placebo group. Such information is usually found in tables in the drugs' package inserts. We also used post-marketing clinical experience as a guide in determining which side effects were common enough to make the list.
- Mechanism of action. While the mechanism of action is not well-established for most psychiatric drugs, we thought it would be important to report the mechanisms most commonly cited.
- Pharmacokinetics, with a focus on drug metabolism and/or half-life.
- Drug interactions.
- Clinical pearls, which typically comment on advantages or disadvantages of a medication in comparison to others in its therapeutic category, tips for dosing or avoiding side effects, types of patients who seem to benefit the most, and so forth.
- Fun facts.
- Lastly, our bottom-line summary or assessment for that particular medication.

PREGNANCY AND LACTATION RISK INFORMATION

The risks and benefits of using psychiatric medications in pregnancy and breastfeeding are not as simple or clear as the previously used "ABCDX" categories might suggest. The new Pregnancy and Lactation Labeling Rule (PLLR) has been implemented by the FDA, resulting in a more detailed narrative describing available risk data instead of the letter category designation. Rather than putting this information in the fact sheets, we have a separate section in the appendix devoted to the topic.

OTHER USEFUL INFORMATION IN THE APPENDICES

Drug interactions in psychiatry. While we do provide some information on drug interactions in the fact sheets, we also have a more extensive discussion of the topic, as well as a table of interactions for commonly prescribed drugs.

Schedules of controlled substances. Just in case you can't remember which drugs are in which DEA schedule or what each schedule means, we have you covered with a handy table. (https://goo.gl/Mo6KEQ).

Lab monitoring for psychiatric medications. We've included a short easy reference table listing the medications that require laboratory monitoring, along with the labs you should consider ordering.

Pharmacogenetic testing recommendations. Although we're not big fans of pharmacogenetic testing, we've added a brief section providing some basic information.

FINANCIAL DISCLOSURES

Dr. Puzantian and Dr. Carlat have disclosed that they have no relevant relationships or financial interests in any commercial company pertaining to the information provided in this book.

DISCLAIMER

The medication information in this book was formulated with a reasonable standard of care and in conformity with professional standards in the field of psychiatry. Medication prescribing decisions are complex, and you should use these fact sheets as only one of many possible sources of medication information. This information is not a substitute for informed medical care. This book is intended for use by licensed professionals only.

If you have any comments or corrections, please let us know by writing to us at info@thecarlatreport.com or *The Carlat Psychiatry Report*, P.O. Box 626, Newburyport, MA 01950.

ADHD Medications

GENERAL PRESCRIBING TIPS

Generally, when you have a patient with ADHD symptoms, your first choice is going to be one of the psychostimulants, because these are usually more effective than the alternatives—atomoxetine, bupropion, and guanfacine. Which psychostimulant will you choose? Here are some of the factors that will influence your decision:

1. *Long-acting vs short-acting.* Choosing between long- and short-acting stimulants is more art than science. Trial and error, combined with patient preference, will dictate the final regimen. Adults will often start with a long-acting agent so they can take a single dose in the morning and have it carry through their workday. Kids may do better with short-acting stimulants so that they will have an appetite when the medication wears off at lunch.
2. *Amphetamine vs methylphenidate.* Generally, this is a Coke vs Pepsi decision—some people like one better than the other, and you can't predict their preference ahead of time. We recommend a methylphenidate over an amphetamine in most cases, because amphetamines tend to have more side effects and are more likely to be abused or diverted.
3. *Stimulants vs non-stimulants.* Stimulants are more effective than non-stimulants, so they are your first-line choice for most patients. If you have a substance abuser, start with atomoxetine. Some special clinical circumstances seem to naturally call for other options. For example, bupropion is helpful for ADHD symptoms, as well as for depression, tobacco use, and being overweight, so it might be a great choice for patients with a combination of these problems. Alpha agonists, such as guanfacine and clonidine, are helpful for both ADHD and insomnia, another potential two-fer, though these meds tend to be used more frequently for children.
4. *Cost.* Most ADHD meds are available generically, but some reasonable choices are still branded and therefore more expensive. The most popular of these is Vyvanse, which is a long-acting amphetamine. Vyvanse appears to have a genuine advantage over many other stimulants, mainly in terms of tolerability and less potential for abuse. However, you'll have a hard time convincing insurance companies to cover the cost of Vyvanse unless you can clearly document intolerance to several other trials of stimulants.

Dose Equivalents

Most patients need to try different stimulants, or stimulant formulations, before settling on the one that works best for them. The dose equivalents are, luckily, fairly easy to remember.

1. From amphetamine to another amphetamine
   - With the exception of Vyvanse, all amphetamines, including both Adderall IR and XR, are roughly equivalent in potency. For example, if a patient is taking Dexedrine 10 mg TID, you can switch this to Adderall 15 BID or Adderall XR 30 mg QD. That said, some people believe that Dexedrine, being 100% dextroamphetamine, might be more potent than Adderall, which is 75% d-amphetamine and 25% l-amphetamine (eg, Dexedrine 30 mg/day may be closer to 40 mg/day of Adderall). In reality, the effect is likely negligible in most people.
   - Vyvanse is composed of both lysine and amphetamine, with amphetamine making up only about 30% of Vyvanse. This means that it's much less potent than straight Dexedrine. So, when switching from another amphetamine to Vyvanse, you have to at least double the dose.
2. From methylphenidate to another methylphenidate
   - With the exception of Concerta and Focalin, all methylphenidate preparations are roughly equivalent in potency.
   - Concerta, because of its complex delivery system, delivers less methylphenidate than implied by the mg amount you prescribe. The usual conversion percentage used is 83%, meaning that the body sees 83% of Concerta in methylphenidate equivalents. Thus, Concerta 18 mg is equivalent to methylphenidate 15 mg, 36 mg is equivalent to 30 mg, and so on.
   - Focalin is the dextro-isomer of methylphenidate, which is twice as potent as methylphenidate. Thus, use about half the dose when prescribing Focalin.
3. From methylphenidate to an amphetamine (or vice versa)
   - Methylphenidate is roughly half as potent as amphetamine, so Ritalin 10 mg = Dexedrine 5 mg, etc. Consistent with this equivalency, child psychiatrists often dose methylphenidate at 1 mg/kg, whereas they dose amphetamine at 0.5 mg/kg. Conversely, if you're switching from Dexedrine to Ritalin, you would need to increase the dose by a factor of two.

How to Switch

Once you've determined the dose equivalence, the actual switching is easy. Don't cross-taper, just have your patient take the last dose of stimulant A on day 1 and start stimulant B on day 2. To be prudent, start the new stimulant at a somewhat lower dose than you calculate would be needed based on the equivalent dose rules of thumb. Those equivalencies are based on averages and may not apply to a given individual.

Side Effects and Class Warnings

The following apply to all stimulants:

- Potential to cause psychosis or aggression: This is a rare and dose-related effect; it may be more likely in patients with a predisposition for psychosis.
- Worsening or new-onset Tourette's or tic disorders: Stimulants may unmask tics. Of stimulants, methylphenidate is favored. The non-stimulant guanfacine is an even better alternative.
- Seizures: Stimulants may lower the seizure threshold, although data are contradictory; monitor patients with seizure disorders closely.
- Growth inhibition or weight loss: With long-term use, some growth inhibition may occur occasionally in children, but this is generally not a major problem. Monitoring growth and considering "drug holidays" may limit growth suppression.
- Cardiovascular safety: The FDA issued a serious class warning in 2006 with regard to cardiovascular safety. However, newer data, both in children and adults, have been reassuring. Cardiac events occurred at virtually the same or lower rates among people who took stimulants compared to those who did not. From a practical perspective, we recommend asking about cardiac problems and consulting the child's pediatrician or cardiologist if a problem exists. Amphetamines should be avoided in patients with known or suspected cardiovascular disease.
- All stimulants are controlled substances, Schedule II, which means they can't be refilled or called in. Patients must be given a new prescription every month. In most states, you are allowed to give patients post-dated prescriptions for convenience.

TABLE 1: ADHD Medications

Brand Name (Generic Name, if different than heading) Year FDA Approved *[G] denotes generic availability*	Available Strengths (mg except where noted)	Usual Dosage Range (starting–max) (mg)	Duration of Action (hours)	Can It Be Split?	Ages Approved for ADHD	Delivery System/Notes (IR = immediate, CR = controlled, DR = delayed release)
Methylphenidates						
Short-acting						
Focalin [G] (Dexmethylphenidate) 2001	2.5, 5, 10	2.5 BID–10 BID	3–4	Yes (not scored)	6–17	Tablet; D-enantiomer of Ritalin; 2x more potent than methylphenidate
Methylin CT [G] 2003	2.5, 5, 10	2.5 BID–20 TID	3–4	Yes	6–17, adults	Chewable, grape-flavored tablet
Methylin oral solution [G] 2002	5 mg/5 mL, 10 mg/5 mL	2.5 BID–20 TID	3–4	N/A	6–17, adults	Clear, grape-flavored liquid
Ritalin [G] 1955	5, 10, 20	2.5 BID–20 TID	3–4	Yes	6–17, adults	IR tablet
Intermediate-acting						
Metadate ER [G] 1999 (Branded generic of Ritalin SR)	20	10 QAM–30 BID	6–8	No	6–17, adults	CR tablet (less predictable because of wax matrix)
Methylin ER [G] 2000 (Branded generic of Ritalin SR)	10, 20	20 QAM–60 QAM	4–8	No	6–17, adults	Hydrophilic polymer tablet; possibly more continuous than others in category
Ritalin SR [G] 1982	10, 20	10 QAM–60 QAM	4–8	No	6–17, adults	CR tablet (less predictable because of wax matrix)
Long-acting						
Aptensio XR 2015	10, 15, 20, 30, 40, 50, 60	10 QAM–60 QAM	8–12	Can be sprinkled; do not crush or chew	6–17, adults	Capsule of 40% IR beads & 60% DR beads
Concerta [G] 2000	18, 27, 36, 54	18 QAM–72 QAM	10–16	No	6–17, adults	CR tablet with 22% IR & 78% DR
Cotempla XR-ODT 2017	8.6, 17.3, 25.9	17.3 QAM–51.8 QAM	8–12	No	6–17	Orally disintegrating, ER with 25% IR & 75% ER
Daytrana patch (Methylphenidate transdermal system) 2006	10, 15, 20, 30	10 QAM–30 QAM. Remove after 9 hours	8–12	No	6–17, adults	CR patch; duration can be shortened by decreasing wear time; drug effects may persist for 5 hours after removal
Focalin XR [G] (Dexmethylphenidate XR) 2005	5, 10, 15, 20, 25, 30, 35, 40	6–17 yrs: 5 QAM–30 QAM; Adults: 10 QAM–40 QAM	8–12	Can be sprinkled; do not crush or chew	6–17, adults	Capsule of 50% IR beads & 50% DR beads; mimics BID dosing; 2x more potent than methylphenidate
Metadate CD [G] 2001	10, 20, 30, 40, 50, 60	20 QAM–60 QAM	8–12	Can be sprinkled; do not crush or chew	6–17, adults	Capsule of 30% IR beads & 70% DR beads; mimics BID dosing
Quillichew ER 2015	20, 30, 40	20 QAM–60 QAM	8–12	Yes	6–17, adults	Chewable ER for those who will not swallow pills or take liquid; 30% IR & 70% ER

Brand Name (Generic Name, if different than heading) Year FDA Approved *[G] denotes generic availability*	Available Strengths (mg except where noted)	Usual Dosage Range (starting–max) (mg)	Duration of Action (hours)	Can It Be Split?	Ages Approved for ADHD	Delivery System/Notes (IR = immediate, CR = controlled, DR = delayed release)
Quillivant XR 2012	25/5 mL	20 QAM–60 QAM	8–12	No	6–17, adults	20% IR & 80% ER in oral solution; shake prior to use
Ritalin LA [G] 2002	10, 20, 30, 40, 60	20 QAM–60 QAM	8–12	Can be sprinkled; do not crush or chew	6–17, adults	Capsule of 50% IR beads & 50% DR beads
Amphetamines						
Short-acting						
Dexedrine [G] (Dextroamphetamine) 1976	5, 10	3–5 yrs: 2.5 QAM–20 BID; 6–16 yrs: 5 QAM–20 BID	3–5	Yes	3–16	Scored tablet
Desoxyn [G] (Methamphetamine) 1943	5	5 QAM–10 BID	3–5	Yes	6–17	Tablet
Evekeo (Amphetamine) 2012	5, 10	3–5 yrs: 2.5 QAM–20 BID; 6–17 yrs: 5 QAM–20 BID	3–5	Yes	3–17	Scored tablet
ProCentra [G] (Dextroamphetamine oral solution) 2008	5 mg/5 mL	5 BID–20 BID	3–5	N/A	3–16	Bubblegum-flavored liquid
Zenzedi (Dextroamphetamine) 2013	2.5, 5, 7.5, 10, 15, 20, 30	3–5 yrs: 2.5 BID–20 BID; 6–16 yrs: 5 QAM–20 BID (same as Dexedrine dosing)	3–5	Yes	3–16	Tablet; 5 mg scored, 10 mg double scored, rest unscored
Intermediate-acting						
Adderall [G] (Mixed amphetamine salts) 1960	5, 7.5, 10, 12.5, 15, 20, 30	3–5 yrs: 2.5 QAM–20 BID; 6–17 yrs: 5 QAM–20 BID; Adults: 5 QAM–20 BID	6–8	Can be crushed	3–17, adults	Tablet; mixed salt of l- and d-amphetamine
Long-acting						
Adderall XR [G] (Mixed amphetamine salts) 2001	5, 10, 15, 20, 25, 30	6–12 yrs: 5 QAM–30 QAM; 13–17 yrs: 10 QAM–40 QAM; Adults: 20 QAM–60 QAM	8–12	Can be sprinkled; do not crush or chew	6–17, adults	Capsule of 50% IR beads & 50% DR beads; mixed salt of l- and d-amphetamine; mimics BID dosing
Adzenys XR-ODT (Amphetamine) 2016	3.1, 6.3, 9.4, 12.5, 15.7, 18.8	6–12 yrs: 6.3 QAM–18.8 QAM; 13–17 yrs: 6.3 QAM–12.5 QAM; Adults: 12.5 QAM	8–12	No (ODT)	6–17, adults	Extended release orally disintegrating tablets; 3.1 mg is equivalent to 5 mg mixed salts product; increasing dose preparations are equivalent to 10 mg, 15 mg, 20 mg, 25 mg, and 30 mg respectively

Brand Name (Generic Name, if different than heading) Year FDA Approved *[G] denotes generic availability*	Available Strengths (mg except where noted)	Usual Dosage Range (starting–max) (mg)	Duration of Action (hours)	Can It Be Split?	Ages Approved for ADHD	Delivery System/Notes (IR = immediate, CR = controlled, DR = delayed release)
Dexedrine Spansules [G] (Dextroamphetamine) 1976	5, 10, 15	5 QAM–20 BID	6–8	Can be sprinkled; do not crush or chew	3–16	Capsule of 50% IR & 50% sustained release beads
Dyanavel XR (Amphetamine) 2015	2.5 mg/mL	6–17 yrs: 2.5 QAM–20 QAM	8–12	No (oral suspension)	6–17	Extended release oral suspension allowing once-daily dosing (must shake well); 2.5 mg = 4 mg mixed amphetamine salts
Mydayis (Mixed amphetamine salts) 2017	12.5, 25, 37.5, 50	13–17 yrs: 12.5 QAM–25 QAM; Adults: 12.5–50 QAM	10–12+	Can be sprinkled; do not crush or chew	13–17, adults	pH-dependent ER capsule formulation; may have effect up to 16 hours
Vyvanse (Lisdexamfetamine) 2007	10, 20, 30, 40, 50, 60, 70	30 QAM–70 QAM	8–12	Can be dissolved in water	6–17, adults	Capsule; chewable tablets also available; lisdexamfetamine is prodrug of dextroamphetamine
Non-Stimulants						
Intuniv (Guanfacine ER) [G] 2009	1, 2, 3, 4	1–4 QD (do not increase faster than 1 mg/wk) (adolescents 7 mg/day max)	24	No	6–17	Extended release tablet; do not stop abruptly (rebound hypertension); not a 1:1 conversion from IR; do not give with high-fat meals
Kapvay [G] (Clonidine XR) 2009	0.1, 0.2	0.1 QHS; increase by 0.1 mg/day weekly and give divided BID; max 0.4 QD	12–16	No	6–17	Extended release tablet; titrate gradually (orthostatic hypotension); avoid abrupt discontinuation; somnolence
Provigil [G] (Modafinil) 1998	100, 200	100 QAM–400 QAM	18–24	Yes (200 mg tabs are scored)	Not FDA-approved for ADHD	Tablet; studies have shown modafinil to be helpful for ADHD, but low incidence of serious rash; minimal data in children
Strattera [G] (Atomoxetine) 2002	10, 18, 25, 40, 60, 80, 100	Dosage varies. See footnote 1 below.	24	No	6–17, adults	Capsule; norepinephrine reuptake inhibitor
Tenex [G] (Guanfacine IR) 1986	1, 2	1–4 QD (do not increase faster than 1 mg/wk)	17	Can be crushed	Not FDA-approved for kids or ADHD. Approved only for adults 18+ for hypertension	Tablet
Wellbutrin [G] (Bupropion) 1985	75, 100	1.4–6 mg/kg/day	6–9	Yes	Not FDA-approved for ADHD	Tablet; bupropion SR & XL versions exist

[1]Strattera dosing: Weight <70kg, start 0.5 mg/kg, target 1.2 mg/kg, max 1.4 mg/kg; weight >70 kg, 40–100 mg

AMPHETAMINE (Adzenys XR-ODT, Dyanavel XR, Evekeo) Fact Sheet

FDA Indications:

ADHD (Adzenys XR-ODT: adults and children ≥6; Dyanavel XR: children ≥6; Evekeo: children ≥3); **narcolepsy** (Evekeo); **obesity** (Evekeo).

Off-Label Uses:

Treatment-resistant depression.

Dosage Forms:

- **Tablets (Evekeo):** 5 mg, 10 mg (scored).
- **ER orally disintegrating tablets (Adzenys XR-ODT):** 3.1 mg, 6.3 mg, 9.4 mg, 12.5 mg, 15.7 mg, 18.8 mg.
- **ER oral suspension (Dyanavel XR):** 2.5 mg/mL.

Dosage Guidance:

- Tablets (Evekeo):
  - Children 3–5: Start 2.5 mg QAM, increase in 2.5 mg/day increments weekly.
  - Children 6–17: Start 5 mg QAM, increase in 5 mg/day increments weekly to maximum of 40 mg/day in divided doses.
  - Narcolepsy: Start 5 mg QAM (ages 6–12) or 10 mg QAM (>12), increase by 5 mg/day or 10 mg/day increments weekly, respectively. Maximum 60 mg/day in divided doses.
- ER ODT (Adzenys XR–ODT):
  - Start 6.3 mg QAM, increase in 3.1–6.3 mg/day increments weekly. Maximum of 18.8 mg/day (ages 6–12) or 12.5 mg/day (ages 13–17 and adults).
- ER oral suspension (Dyanavel XR):
  - Children 6–12: Start 2.5 mg–5 mg QAM, increase in 2.5 mg–10 mg/day increments every 4–7 days. Maximum 20 mg/day.

Monitoring: ECG if history of cardiac disease.

Cost: $$$$

Side Effects:

- Most common: Abdominal pain, decreased appetite, weight loss, insomnia, headache, nervousness.
- Serious but rare: See class warnings in chapter introduction.

Mechanism, Pharmacokinetics, and Drug Interactions:

- Stimulant that inhibits reuptake of dopamine and norepinephrine.
- Metabolized primarily via CYP2D6; t ½: 11 hours.
- Avoid use with MAOIs, antacids.

Clinical Pearls:

- These racemic forms of amphetamine differ from dextroamphetamine in that the l-isomer component is more potent than the d-isomer in peripheral activity (potentially resulting in more cardiovascular effects, tics).
- There may be less appetite suppressant effects with a racemic mixture compared to dextroamphetamine.
- Divide IR (Evekeo) doses by 4–6 hour intervals.
- Approximate equivalence doses of Adzenys XR-ODT and mixed amphetamine salts XR (Adderall XR) are: 3.1 mg = 5 mg, 6.3 mg = 10 mg, 9.4 mg = 15 mg, 12.5 mg = 20 mg, 15.7 mg = 25 mg, 18.8 mg = 30 mg.
- Dyanavel XR is an oral suspension. Shake well to get the intended extended release effect. The approximate equivalence of 2.5 mg/mL is 4 mg of mixed amphetamine salts.

Fun Fact:

The term "amphetamine" is the contracted form of the chemical "alpha-methylphenethylamine." Its first pharmacologic use was when pharmaceutical company Smith, Kline and French sold amphetamine under the trade name Benzedrine as a decongestant inhaler.

Bottom Line:

Newer formulations of an old drug come with a high price tag. Stick to the usual amphetamine products like mixed amphetamine salts unless liquid or ODT dosing is absolutely necessary.

ATOMOXETINE (Strattera) Fact Sheet [G]

FDA Indications:

ADHD (adults and children ≥6 years).

Off-Label Uses:

Treatment-resistant depression.

Dosage Forms:

Capsules (G): 10 mg, 18 mg, 25 mg, 40 mg, 60 mg, 80 mg, 100 mg.

Dosage Guidance:

- Start 40 mg QAM for 3 days, ↑ to 80 mg QAM, may ↑ to 100 mg/day after 2–4 weeks if needed (max 100 mg/day); may divide doses >40 mg/day (morning and late afternoon/early evening).
- Special dosing for children <70 kg:
  Start 0.5 mg/kg QAM for 3 days, ↑ to 1.2 mg/kg QAM, may ↑ to max 1.4 mg/kg/day or 100 mg/day (whichever is less) after 2–4 weeks, if needed; may divide doses >0.5 mg/kg/day.

Monitoring: Baseline LFTs, follow up if signs of liver disease.

Cost: $$$

Side Effects:

- Most common: *Children:* Headache, abdominal pain, decreased appetite, fatigue, nausea, vomiting.
  Adults: Nausea, dry mouth, decreased appetite, insomnia, constipation, fatigue, erectile dysfunction, abdominal pain, dizziness, urinary hesitation.
- Serious but rare: Class warning for suicidal ideation in children and teens. Severe hepatic injury including increased hepatic enzymes (up to 40 times normal) and jaundice (bilirubin up to 12 times upper limit of normal). Increased blood pressure (↑ 15–20 mmHg) and heart rate (↑ 20 bpm).

Mechanism, Pharmacokinetics, and Drug Interactions:

- Selective norepinephrine reuptake inhibitor (NRI).
- Metabolized primarily via CYP2D6; t ½: 5 hours.
- Avoid use with MAOIs. Exercise caution with 2D6 inhibitors such as fluoxetine, paroxetine, and quinidine (increased atomoxetine serum levels); use slower titration and do not exceed 80 mg/day in presence of 2D6 inhibitors or in 2D6 poor metabolizers.

Clinical Pearls:

- QAM dosing is as effective as BID, but BID dosing has better GI tolerability. Can also be dosed at bedtime if it causes fatigue.
- Appears to be more effective in improving attention than in controlling hyperactivity.
- Labs: Order baseline liver function tests.

Fun Fact:

Atomoxetine was originally known as "tomoxetine"; however, the FDA requested that the name be changed because the similarity to "tamoxifen" could lead to dispensing errors.

Bottom Line:

- *Advantages:* Unlike stimulants, atomoxetine carries no abuse potential, causes less insomnia and anxiety, and is unlikely to worsen tics.
- *Disadvantages:* Generally less effective than stimulants, and takes longer to work (2–4 weeks).

DEXMETHYLPHENIDATE (Focalin) Fact Sheet [G]

FDA Indications:
ADHD in adults (XR only) and in children ≥6 years (IR and XR).

Off-Label Uses:
Narcolepsy, obesity, treatment-resistant depression.

Dosage Forms:
- **Tablets (G):** 2.5 mg, 5 mg, 10 mg.
- **ER capsules (G):** 5 mg, 10 mg, 15 mg, 20 mg, 25 mg, 30 mg, 35 mg, 40 mg.

Dosage Guidance:
- IR: Start 2.5 mg BID, ↑ by 5 mg–10 mg/day every 7 days. Max 20 mg/day; divide IR doses by at least 4 hours.
- ER: Start 10 mg QAM, ↑ by 10 mg/day every 7 days. Max 40 mg/day. For children, start 5 mg QAM, ↑ by 5 mg/day every 7 days. Max (children) 30 mg/day.

Monitoring: ECG if history of cardiac disease.

Cost: IR: $; ER: $$$

Side Effects:
- Most common: Decreased appetite, insomnia, anxiety, GI distress, irritability, tics, headache, tachycardia, hypertension, dry mouth.
- Serious but rare: See cardiovascular class warning in chapter introduction.

Mechanism, Pharmacokinetics, and Drug Interactions:
- Stimulant that inhibits reuptake of dopamine and norepinephrine.
- Metabolized primarily via de-esterification, not CYP450; t ½: 2–4.5 hours (2–3 hours in children); ER delivers 50% of dose immediately and 50% about 5 hours later.
- Avoid use with MAOIs.

Clinical Pearls:
- Focalin is the d-isomer of methylphenidate and is 2x more potent than methylphenidate, which is why it is prescribed at about half the dose.
- Use the same total daily dose of Focalin IR as Focalin XR.
- Focalin XR capsules contain two kinds of beads: Half are immediate release beads and half are enteric coated delayed release beads. A single, once-daily dose of XR capsule provides the same amount of dexmethylphenidate as 2 IR tablets given 4 hours apart.
- The ER capsules cannot be split in half. However, they can be opened and the beads sprinkled over food. The patient should then eat all that food—eating half won't work to split the dose accurately because it won't be possible to determine if the eaten portion contains more immediate release or delayed release beads.
- Give with food if GI side effects occur.

Fun Fact:
With 2 stereoactive centers, methylphenidate has 4 possible stereoisomers. Of the 4, dexmethylphenidate is the most active biologically.

Bottom Line:
Focalin is just Ritalin but more potent. It's available as a generic and may mean fewer tablets for patients. Focalin XR only recently went generic, so it will likely remain quite expensive for a while.

DEXTROAMPHETAMINE (Dexedrine) Fact Sheet [G]

FDA Indications:
ADHD (children ≥3 years); **narcolepsy** (adults and children ≥6 years).

Off-Label Uses:
Obesity, treatment-resistant depression.

Dosage Forms:
- **Tablets (Dexedrine) (G):** 5 mg, 10 mg (scored).
- **Tablets (Zenzedi):** 2.5 mg, 5 mg, 7.5 mg, 10 mg, 15 mg, 20 mg, 30 mg (5 mg scored, 10 mg double scored; rest unscored).
- **ER capsules (Dexedrine Spansules) (G):** 5 mg, 10 mg, 15 mg.
- **Liquid (ProCentra) (G):** 5 mg/5 mL.

Dosage Guidance:
- ADHD (IR and ER):
  - Adults and children ≥6 years: Start 5 mg QAM, ↑ by 5 mg/day at weekly intervals to max 60 mg/day though doses ≥40 mg/day are rarely more effective. Divide IR dose QD–TID.
  - Children 3–5 years: Start 2.5 mg QAM, ↑ by 2.5 mg/day weekly to max 60 mg/day though doses >40 mg/day are rarely more effective. Divide IR dose QD–TID.
- Narcolepsy (IR and ER):
  - Start 10 mg QAM, ↑ by 10 mg/day weekly to max 60 mg/day. Divide IR dose QD–TID.

Monitoring: ECG if history of cardiac disease.

Cost: IR: $$ (Zenzedi and ProCentra: $$$$); ER: $$$

Side Effects:
- Most common: Abdominal pain, anorexia, nausea, tics, insomnia, tachycardia, and headache.
- Serious but rare: See class warnings in chapter introduction.

Mechanism, Pharmacokinetics, and Drug Interactions:
- Stimulant that inhibits reuptake of dopamine and norepinephrine.
- Metabolized primarily through CYP450 2D6 (minor) and glucuronidation; t ½: 12 hours.
- Avoid use with MAOIs, antacids.

Clinical Pearls:
- Dextroamphetamine is the more potent d-isomer of amphetamine; it has potentially less peripheral effects (eg, motor tics) than a racemic mix (eg, mixed amphetamine salts like Adderall, amphetamine, or methamphetamine).
- IR tablets and oral solution: Doses can be given at intervals of 4–6 hours.
- Dextroamphetamine is the only stimulant, other than Adderall IR, approved for children <6 years (approved for children ≥3 years).
- The new Zenzedi brand offers more dosing flexibility options, but it is more expensive than generic IR tablets.
- Also available as D,L racemic mixture of amphetamine as Evekeo tablets, Adzenys XR-ODT, and as Dyanavel XR oral suspension (see amphetamine fact sheet).

Fun Fact:
Dexys Midnight Runners, the British band famous for its song "Come On Eileen" (1982), derived their name from Dexedrine—"Dexys" after the drug's name and "Midnight Runners" in reference to the energy it provides.

Bottom Line:
Good drug, with very long history of experience, available in short- and long-acting formulations as generics.

GUANFACINE (Intuniv, Tenex) Fact Sheet [G]

FDA Indications:
ADHD (children ages 6–17), as monotherapy or adjunctive therapy to stimulants (not approved for ADHD in adults).

Off-Label Uses:
Conduct disorder; Tourette's and motor tics; pervasive developmental disorders; migraine prophylaxis; opioid withdrawal.

Dosage Forms:
- **IR tablets (Tenex, G):** 1 mg, 2 mg.
- **ER tablets (Intuniv, G):** 1 mg, 2 mg, 3 mg, 4 mg.

Dosage Guidance:
- IR dosing depends on weight.
  - 27 kg–40.5 kg (55–90 lbs): Start 0.5 mg QHS, ↑ by 0.5 mg/day at weekly intervals up to 1.5 mg/day, may ↑ to 2 mg/day after 2 weeks; max 2 mg/day in 2 to 4 divided doses.
  - 40.5 kg–45 kg (90–99 lbs): Start 0.5 mg QHS, ↑ by 0.5 mg/day at weekly intervals; max 1 mg per dose, 3 mg/day.
  - >45 kg (>99 lbs): Start 1 mg QHS, ↑ by 1 mg/day at weekly intervals up to 3 mg/day, may ↑ to 4 mg/day after 2 weeks; max 1 mg per dose, 4 mg/day.
- ER: Start 1 mg QHS, ↑ by 1 mg/day at weekly intervals; max 4 mg/day. Alternative: 0.05 mg/kg–0.12 mg/kg QD or QHS; max 4 mg/day. Doses up to 7 mg/day ER studied as monotherapy in adolescents.

Monitoring: Blood pressure.

Cost: IR: $; ER: $

Side Effects:
- Most common: Dry mouth, somnolence, dizziness, constipation, fatigue, headache.
- Serious but rare: Hypotension, syncope, orthostasis.

Mechanism, Pharmacokinetics, and Drug Interactions:
- Centrally-acting, selective alpha-2 adrenergic agonist.
- Metabolized primarily through CYP3A4; t ½: 13–14 hours in children (16–18 in adults).
- Avoid use with MAOIs. Caution with 3A4 inhibitors (eg, clarithromycin, fluvoxamine) and inducers (eg, St. John's wort, carbamazepine).

Clinical Pearls:
- Not a controlled substance.
- Guanfacine IR and ER are not interchangeable on a mg:mg basis. When switching from one formulation to the other, taper and retitrate.
- Guanfacine tends to be less sedating than clonidine, another alpha agonist.
- If patient misses 2 or more consecutive doses, consider repeating titration.
- ER tablets should not be taken with a high-fat meal due to increased medication exposure.
- Minimize side effects, especially somnolence, by administering at bedtime.
- Monitor blood pressure, especially during initial dosing titration.
- Risk of nervousness, anxiety, and possibly rebound hypertension 2–4 days after abrupt discontinuation. Taper dose in 1 mg/day decrements, every 3–7 days.

Fun Fact:
Some prescribers have taken advantage of guanfacine's sympatholytic properties for the treatment of nightmares and dissociative symptoms in PTSD.

Bottom Line:
Advantages over stimulants include no worsening of tic disorders, lack of abuse potential, and no insomnia. However, its delayed onset of effect (2–4 weeks) and lower efficacy rates make it a second-line choice for ADHD generally. ER is now available in generic and easier to use than IR.

LISDEXAMFETAMINE (Vyvanse) Fact Sheet

FDA Indications:

ADHD (adults and children ≥6 years); **binge eating disorder** (BED).

Off-Label Uses:

Narcolepsy; obesity; treatment-resistant depression.

Dosage Forms:

- **Capsules:** 10 mg, 20 mg, 30 mg, 40 mg, 50 mg, 60 mg, 70 mg.
- **Chewtabs:** 10 mg, 20 mg, 30 mg, 40 mg, 50 mg, 60 mg.

Dosage Guidance:

- ADHD (adults and children ≥6 years): Start 30 mg QAM, ↑ by 10 mg–20 mg/day at weekly intervals. Target lowest effective dose; max 70 mg/day.
- BED: Start 30 mg QAM, ↑ by 20 mg/day at weekly intervals to target 50 mg/day; max 70 mg/day.

Monitoring: ECG if history of cardiac disease.

Cost: $$$$

Side Effects:

- Most common: Headache, insomnia, anorexia, abdominal pain, irritability, agitation, tics, decreased appetite, increased heart rate, jitteriness, anxiety.
- Serious but rare: See class warnings in chapter introduction.

Mechanism, Pharmacokinetics, and Drug Interactions:

- Stimulant that inhibits reuptake of dopamine and norepinephrine.
- Metabolized primarily through non-CYP-mediated hepatic and/or intestinal metabolism; t ½: lisdexamfetamine (inactive prodrug) <1 hour; dextroamphetamine (active metabolite) 12 hours. Dextroamphetamine metabolized by CYP2D6.
- Avoid use with MAOIs and antacids. Caution with antihypertensives (decreased efficacy of antihypertensive). Caution with 2D6 inhibitors, which may increase stimulant effects.

Clinical Pearls:

- Lisdexamfetamine is dextroamphetamine with the chemical lysine bound to it, which renders it inactive. It remains inactive until GI enzymes cleave off lysine and convert it to active dextroamphetamine. This means that drug abusers can't get high by snorting it or injecting it.
- Anecdotally, Vyvanse has a more gradual onset and offset than other stimulants, and may cause fewer side effects than other amphetamines.
- Taking with food decreases the effect slightly and delays peak levels by an hour. If patients feel it's not "kicking in" fast enough, have them take it earlier or on an empty stomach.
- Lisdexamfetamine 70 mg is equivalent to 30 mg of mixed amphetamine salts (Adderall).
- While indicated for BED, it is not approved for use as a weight loss or anti-obesity agent.

Fun Fact:

The manufacturer of Vyvanse pursued an indication as an add-on medication for depression, but disappointing results in clinical trials put an end to this effort.

Bottom Line:

Vyvanse may have a gentler, "smoother" side effect profile than other amphetamines, and probably has a lower risk of diversion or abuse. However, its high cost means insurance companies don't like to pay for it without prior authorizations.

METHAMPHETAMINE (Desoxyn) Fact Sheet [G]

FDA Indications:
ADHD (children ≥6 years); **obesity** (adults and adolescents ≥12 years).

Dosage Forms:
Tablets (G): 5 mg.

Dosage Guidance:
ADHD (adults and children ≥6 years): Start 5 mg QAM–BID, ↑ by 5 mg/day at weekly intervals to max 20 mg/day, divided BID.

Monitoring: ECG if history of cardiac disease.

Cost: $$$$

Side Effects:
- Most common: Anorexia, tachycardia, dizziness, insomnia, tremor, tics, restlessness, headache, constipation (decreased GI motility). Dental complications, such as poor dental hygiene, diffuse cavities, bruxism, and tooth wear, may develop with abuse.
- Serious but rare: See class warnings in chapter introduction.

Mechanism, Pharmacokinetics, and Drug Interactions:
- Stimulant that inhibits reuptake of dopamine and norepinephrine.
- Metabolized primarily through CYP2D6 to active metabolite (amphetamine); t ½: 4–5 hours.
- Avoid use with MAOIs and antacids. Caution with 2D6 inhibitors, which may increase stimulant effects.

Clinical Pearls:
- High risk of abuse.
- Not widely used (DEA reports that there were only 16,000 prescriptions written in 2012). When prescribed for obesity, the recommendation is for short-term (ie, a few weeks) use only and as an adjunct to caloric restriction due to its high addiction and diversion potential.
- CNS stimulating effect is approximately equal to or greater than that of amphetamine but less than that of dextroamphetamine; less blood pressure elevation than with amphetamine.

Fun Facts:
Desoxyn is the same as the abused street drug methamphetamine, just pharmaceutical grade. Although methamphetamine and amphetamine were long thought to be available only via laboratories, methamphetamine has been reported to occur naturally in certain acacia trees that grow in West Texas.

Bottom Line:
Highly addictive substance; its use is generally not recommended. Watch the television show "Breaking Bad" if you're not convinced!

METHYLPHENIDATE IR (Ritalin) Fact Sheet [G]

FDA Indications:
ADHD (adults and children ≥6 years); **narcolepsy**.

Off-Label Uses:
Obesity; treatment-resistant depression.

Dosage Forms:
- **Tablets (G):** 5 mg, 10 mg, 20 mg.
- **Chewable tablets (G):** 2.5 mg, 5 mg, 10 mg.
- **Oral solution (G):** 5 mg/5 mL, 10 mg/5 mL.

Dosage Guidance:
- ADHD:
  - Adults: Start 5 mg–10 mg BID, ↑ by 10 mg/day at weekly intervals to max 60 mg/day.
  - Children ≥6 years: Start 0.3 mg/kg BID or 2.5 mg–5 mg BID before breakfast and lunch, increase by 0.1 mg/kg/dose or 5 mg–10 mg/day at weekly intervals to a max of 2 mg/kg/day or 60 mg/day.
- Narcolepsy: Same dosing as ADHD.

Monitoring: ECG if history of cardiac disease.

Cost: $; chewable tabs, oral solution: $$$

Side Effects:
- Most common: Insomnia, headache, nervousness, abdominal pain, nausea, vomiting, anorexia, weight loss, affect lability, tics.
- Serious but rare: See class warnings in chapter introduction.

Mechanism, Pharmacokinetics, and Drug Interactions:
- Stimulant that inhibits reuptake of dopamine and norepinephrine.
- Hepatic metabolism via carboxylesterase CES1A1, not CYP450 isoenzymes; t ½: 2–4 hours.
- Avoid use with MAOIs, antacids.

Clinical Pearls:
- Methylphenidate generally causes fewer side effects than amphetamine preparations—patients are less likely to report feeling "wired."
- While all stimulants may cause tics, a Cochrane review of 8 randomized trials showed that methylphenidate did not worsen tics in children with ADHD and a tic disorder; in some cases it even improved tics.
- Methylin chewable tablet: Administer with at least 8 ounces of water or other fluid.

Fun Fact:
Methylphenidate was synthesized by Ciba (now Novartis) chemist Leandro Panizzon. His wife, Marguerite, had low blood pressure and would take the stimulant before playing tennis. He named the substance "Ritaline" (yes, with the "e" on the end) after his wife's nickname, Rita.

Bottom Line:
Better side effect profile and somewhat lower abuse potential than amphetamines. However, patients often prefer the "kick" they get from Adderall.

METHYLPHENIDATE ER (Concerta, Ritalin SR and LA) Fact Sheet [G]

FDA Indications:
ADHD (adults and children ≥6 years); **narcolepsy**.

Off-Label Uses:
Obesity; treatment-resistant depression.

Dosage Forms (more commonly used):
- **SR tablets (Ritalin SR, Metadate ER, Methylin ER) (G):** 10 mg, 20 mg.
- **ER capsules (Ritalin LA) (G):** 10 mg, 20 mg, 30 mg, 40 mg, 60 mg (50% IR/50% ER).
- **ER capsules (Metadate CD) (G):** 10 mg, 20 mg, 30 mg, 40 mg, 50 mg, 60 mg (30% IR/70% ER).
- **ER capsules (Aptensio XR):** 10 mg, 15 mg, 20 mg, 30 mg, 40 mg, 50 mg, 60 mg (40% IR/60% ER).
- **ER tablets (Concerta) (G):** 18 mg, 27 mg, 36 mg, 54 mg (22% IR/78% ER).
- **ER oral suspension (Quillivant XR):** 25 mg/5 mL (20% IR/80% ER).
- **ER chewable tablets (Quillichew ER):** 20 mg, 30 mg, 40 mg (30% IR/70% ER).
- **ER orally disintegrating tablets (Cotempla):** 8.6 mg, 17.3 mg, 25.9 mg (25% IR/75% ER).

Dosage Guidance:
- Intermediate-acting (Ritalin SR, Metadate ER, Methylin ER):
  - Titrate to effective daily dose with IR, then switch to equivalent 8-hour SR or ER dose QAM–BID (eg, 20 mg ER QAM or BID); max 60 mg/day.
- Long-acting (Aptensio XR, Metadate CD, Ritalin LA, Quillivant XR):
  - Start 20 mg QAM, ↑ by 10 mg–20 mg/day at weekly intervals; max 60 mg/day.
- Long-acting (Cotempla):
  - Start 17.3 mg QAM, ↑ by 8.6–17.3 mg/day at weekly intervals; max 51.8 mg/day.
  - 8.6 mg, 17.3 mg, 25.9 mg equivalent to 10 mg, 20 mg, 30 mg of other methylphenidate formulations, respectively.
- Long-acting (Concerta):
  - Start 18 mg–36 mg QAM, ↑ by 18 mg/day at weekly intervals; max 72 mg/day.
  - Children ≥6 years: start 18 mg QAM, ↑ by 18 mg/day in weekly intervals to max 54 mg/day (ages 6–12) or 72 mg/day (age 13+).
  - If switching from different form of methylphenidate:
    - 10 mg–15 mg/day: Use 18 mg QAM.
    - 20 mg–30 mg/day: Use 36 mg QAM.
    - 30 mg–45 mg/day: Use 54 mg QAM.
    - 40 mg–60 mg/day: Use 72 mg QAM.
    - 27 mg dose is available for situations in which a dose between 18 mg–36 mg is desired.
- Narcolepsy: Start 10 mg–20 mg ER QAM, ↑ by 10 mg/day at weekly intervals; max 60 mg/day.

Monitoring: ECG if history of cardiac disease.

Cost: $$$; Aptensio XR, Quillivant XR, Quillichew ER: $$$$

Side Effects and Mechanism, Pharmacokinetics, and Drug Interactions:
See methylphenidate IR fact sheet.

Clinical Pearls:
- **ER capsules** contain a mixture of 30% IR and 70% ER beads. **Aptensio XR,** a new branded formulation of ER capsules, contains a mixture of 40% IR and 60% ER beads. **Ritalin LA** and its generic ER capsules are a combination of 50% IR and 50% DR beads. These products mimic BID dosing of IR.
- **Cotempla** delivers a mixture of 25% IR and 75% ER in an orally disintegrating extended release formulation.
- **Concerta** is based on the OROS osmotic delivery system (also used for Invega). 22% of dose is immediate (with effects in 1–2 hours) and 78% is delayed.
- To avoid insomnia, dosing of these formulations should be completed by noon.
- **ER** capsules may be opened and contents sprinkled onto small amount (1 tablespoon) of cold applesauce (swallow without chewing).

Bottom Line:
There are many longer-acting methylphenidate preparations. Two good options are Concerta and Ritalin LA, both of which are now available generically.

METHYLPHENIDATE TRANSDERMAL (Daytrana) Fact Sheet

FDA Indications:
ADHD (adults and children ≥6 years).

Dosage Forms:
Transdermal patch: 10 mg, 15 mg, 20 mg, 30 mg/9 hour.

Dosage Guidance:
Start 10 mg/9 hour patch QAM (for initial therapy or for patients switching from other methylphenidate preparations, regardless of dose). Apply to hip 2 hours before an effect is needed and remove 9 hours after application (drug effects may persist for 5 hours after removal). Increase dose at weekly intervals by using next higher dose system. May be removed in <9 hours if shorter duration is desired or if late-day side effects occur. Rotate application sites. Max 30 mg QD.

Monitoring: ECG if history of cardiac disease.

Cost: $$$$

Side Effects:
- Most common: Headache, insomnia, irritability, decreased appetite, anorexia, nausea, tics, application site reaction (10%–40% incidence in children).
- Serious but rare: Allergic contact dermatitis/sensitization, characterized by intense local reactions (eg, edema, papules) that may spread beyond patch site; sensitization may subsequently manifest systemically with other routes of methylphenidate administration.

Mechanism, Pharmacokinetics, and Drug Interactions:
- Stimulant that inhibits reuptake of dopamine and norepinephrine.
- Hepatic metabolism via carboxylesterase CES1A1, not CYP450 isoenzymes; t ½: 3–4 hours.
- Avoid use with MAOIs, antacids.

Clinical Pearls:
- Apply patch to clean, dry area of the hip; don't apply to waistline or to areas under tight clothes, as it may rub off. Alternate sites daily (eg, opposite hip). Absorption not affected by perspiration. Remove after 9 hours. If dislodged, replace with a new patch but remove within the 9-hour total wear time.
- Clinical effect usually seen in 2 hours and lasts approximately 12 hours.
- Exposure of application site to a heat source (eg, hair dryer, heating pad, electric blanket) may increase the amount of drug absorbed.
- In June 2015, the FDA added a warning that Daytrana could cause chemical leukoderma, a permanent loss of skin color. These reactions are irreversible and not harmful but can be disfiguring to patients. Instruct patients to contact their physician if they notice skin color changes or lightening of skin areas; in such cases an alternative medication should be considered.

Fun Fact:
Since 2006, Shire Pharmaceuticals has issued at least 10 recalls of Daytrana patches because users have had difficulty removing the protective cover from the patch. Recall costs have reached into the millions.

Bottom Line:
Daytrana is helpful for kids who, for whatever reason, cannot use any of the wide variety of oral stimulant preparations. Otherwise, we don't recommend it due to high cost, lag time for onset of effect, and the side effect of rash, which is pretty common and unpleasant.

MIXED AMPHETAMINE SALTS (Adderall) Fact Sheet [G]

FDA Indications:
ADHD (adults and children ≥3 years for IR, ≥6 years for XR, ≥13 years for Mydayis); **narcolepsy** (adults and children ≥6 years).

Off-Label Uses:
Obesity; treatment-resistant depression.

Dosage Forms:
- **Tablets (G):** 5 mg, 7.5 mg, 10 mg, 12.5 mg, 15 mg, 20 mg, 30 mg.
- **ER capsules (G):** 5 mg, 10 mg, 15 mg, 20 mg, 25 mg, 30 mg.
- **ER capsules (Mydayis):** 12.5 mg, 25 mg, 37.5 mg, 50 mg.

Dosage Guidance:
- ADHD
  - Rule of thumb for both preparations: Initial dose should be 0.5 mg/kg, but shoot for a target dose of 1.0 mg/kg–1.2 mg/kg.
  - Adults:
    - IR: Start 5 QAM–BID, max 40 mg/day divided BID.
    - ER: Start 20 mg QAM, increase to max 60 mg/day QAM. For Mydayis, start 12.5 mg QAM, increase in increments of 12.5 mg/day weekly, to max 50 mg/day.
  - Children and adolescents:
    - IR: Start 2.5 mg–5 mg BID, max 40 mg/day divided BID.
    - ER: Start 5 mg–10 mg QAM, increase gradually to max 30 mg/day, or 40 mg/day QAM in adolescents. For Mydayis (adolescents ≥13 years), start 12.5 mg QAM, increase in increments of 12.5 mg/day weekly, to max 25 mg/day.
- Narcolepsy: Start 10 mg QAM, increase by 10 mg/day at weekly increments; max 60 mg/day.

Monitoring: ECG if history of cardiac disease.

Cost: IR: $; ER: $$$

Side Effects:
- Most common: Insomnia, headache, decreased appetite, abdominal pain, weight loss, agitation.
- Serious but rare: See class warnings in chapter introduction.

Mechanism, Pharmacokinetics, and Drug Interactions:
- Stimulant that inhibits reuptake of dopamine and norepinephrine.
- Metabolized primarily through CYP2D6; t ½: 9–14 hours. Duration of action: 6–8 hours (IR), 8–12 hours (XR).
- Avoid use with MAOIs, antacids. Caution with 2D6 inhibitors, which may increase stimulant effects.

Clinical Pearls:
- Each dose contains a mixture of amphetamine salts, resulting in a 75:25 ratio of dextro and levo isomers of amphetamine.
- When converting from IR to ER, use the same total daily dose, given QAM.
- Adderall may provide more of a "kick" than methylphenidate preparations. Roughly twice as potent (per mg) as methylphenidate.
- Mydayis is formulated with pH-dependent drug-releasing beads, with immediate release beads and delayed release beads that release drug at pH 5.5 and pH 7.0. Duration of effect may be up to 16 hours.
- Dextroamphetamine and mixed amphetamine salts are the only stimulants approved for children <6 years (approved for children ≥3 years), with the exception of Mydayis, which causes very high rates of side effects (insomnia, reduced appetite) in children <13 years and should only be used in children ≥13 years.

Fun Fact:
Was briefly pulled from the market in Canada in 2005 because of cardiac concerns.

Bottom Line:
Adderall is effective but is probably the most abused and diverted of all stimulants, which is why we recommend starting most patients on methylphenidate instead.

Antidepressants

GENERAL PRESCRIBING TIPS

It's particularly hard to suggest a first-line antidepressant prescription because antidepressants are effective for so many other conditions. Nonetheless, it is helpful to review the most common clinical scenarios:

Medication-Naïve Patients with "Just" Depression

For these patients (admittedly unusual in a psychiatric practice), you want something effective and with minimal side effects. This means either an SSRI or bupropion. While most of us start with an SSRI, we recommend considering bupropion as your go-to first-line agent. With bupropion, you get an effective antidepressant with essentially no sexual side effects, no weight gain, no sedation, and a boost in attention. While it has not been approved for any anxiety disorders, bupropion is just as effective as SSRIs for the nonspecific anxiety that usually accompanies depression. On the downside, you have potential insomnia, and a small risk of seizure—but only at doses above 300 mg/day.

If you start with an SSRI, go with escitalopram or sertraline. Both have minimal side effects and minimal drug-drug interactions.

Patients Who Have Comorbid Conditions

Patients with depression plus another psychiatric disorder can be tried on "twofer" meds—that is, antidepressants that have clear efficacy for two conditions. Here are some of the common secondary conditions and meds that are effective for them: anxiety disorders (TCAs, SSRIs), bulimia (fluoxetine), smoking cessation (bupropion), ADHD (bupropion), fibromyalgia (duloxetine), diabetic neuropathic pain (duloxetine), and premenstrual dysphoric disorder (SSRIs). Finally, mirtazapine—an antidepressant sometimes shunned because it causes weight gain—is an excellent choice for patients with depression who are underweight and have insomnia, and has the benefit of no sexual side effects.

Patients Who Have Been on Other Antidepressants

"Treatment-resistant depression" is usually defined as the failure of at least two prior trials of antidepressants at adequate doses and for adequate lengths of time. Such patients fall into two classes: those who have failed the antidepressants on someone else's watch, and those who have failed them on your watch. When a new patient gives you a list of antidepressants that have already been tried, you have a judgment call to make. Some patients may seem more reliable than others, but on the other hand, you may want to obtain records from prior treatment that are credible.

If the patient fails some antidepressants that you prescribed, you can be more confident of a diagnosis of treatment-resistant depression. There's unfortunately no convincing data on what your next step should be. The Star-D trial tried to tease out strategies such as switching vs augmenting, but it could not find statistical differences between the techniques. That means we're left with a combination of the few clinical trials that have been published, leavened with a great deal of personal preference. Here's a reasonable approach:

- First, try switching to an antidepressant in a different class. Assuming the treatment failures were on SSRIs, the usual sequence of subsequent trials would be: 1) bupropion or mirtazapine; 2) an SNRI (venlafaxine, duloxetine, levomilnacipran); 3) an MAOI or a tricyclic. The usual technique for switching antidepressants is to do a cross-taper/titration, in which you gradually increase the dose of the new medication while decreasing the dose of the old one. This strategy is especially important when the med to be stopped is known to cause discontinuation symptoms (see below). Abrupt switches are probably fine when moving from one SSRI to another—unless you are stopping paroxetine, which is highly likely to cause discontinuation reactions and should be gradually tapered.
- Second, try a combination. A suggested order of combinations to try is: 1) SSRI/SNRI + bupropion; 2) SSRI/SNRI + atypical antipsychotic; 3) SSRI/SNRI + lithium or thyroid supplementation. There are many more combination possibilities, but these are probably the highest yield with which to begin.
- Third, hit the neurostimulation devices, such as ECT, TMS, and others.

Class Warnings

There are some side effects or warnings that apply to **all** antidepressants. They are listed here in order to minimize repetition in the fact sheets that follow.

Suicide risk

A black box warning regarding an increased risk of suicidal ideation in children and adolescents was added to the labeling on all antidepressants by the FDA in 2004. The warning was based on retrospective reports that showed a very slight increase in suicidal ideation in patients on 9 different antidepressants. The warning was revised in 2007 to also include adolescents and young adults, up to age 24. Since then, more prospective data have emerged that do not support an association, and this warning has been called further into question. In fact, the data suggest that severity of depression itself is associated with increased risk of suicide.

For now, however, the warning remains and is applied to the labeling of all medications approved for the treatment of depression. Thus, you should monitor all patients closely—especially early in therapy or after medication discontinuation—for clinical worsening, changes in behavior, or suicidality.

Mania switch

Activation of mania or hypomania may occur with the use of any antidepressant in individuals who are at risk. Antidepressants should be used with caution in patients with a history of mania or hypomania, or in those with a family history of bipolar disorder.

Serotonin syndrome

A rare but potentially life-threatening condition called serotonin syndrome (agitation, hallucinations, other mental status changes, hyperthermia, tachycardia, labile BP, myoclonus, hyperreflexia, incoordination, nausea, vomiting, diarrhea) has been reported when serotonergic antidepressants have been used with other serotonergic agents (including SSRIs, SNRIs, buspirone, lithium, MAOIs).

Discontinuation syndrome

Abrupt discontinuation of antidepressants, particularly SSRIs and SNRIs, may result in a discontinuation syndrome. While not medically dangerous and generally self-limiting, the syndrome may be uncomfortable for patients. Symptoms include dizziness, nausea, headache, irritability, insomnia, diarrhea, agitation, sensory disturbances (eg, electric shock sensations), lethargy, and abnormal dreams. In general, symptoms are more severe with higher-dose and longer-term antidepressant use. Agents that are particularly short-acting may have a higher likelihood of causing a discontinuation syndrome (eg, paroxetine, venlafaxine IR) compared to longer-acting agents (eg, fluoxetine). In cases of planned discontinuation, antidepressant dose should be gradually reduced.

Bleeding risk

Increased bleeding episodes (eg, GI bleed, bruising, nosebleed) have been reported with serotonergic antidepressants, particularly when they are used concomitantly with aspirin, NSAIDs, anticoagulants, or antiplatelet agents. Occasionally, surgeons will request that patients stop SSRIs before surgery in order to decrease the bleeding risk. While this practice does not reflect the standard of care, it might be reasonable in situations where the risk of bleeding is especially high.

TABLE 2: Antidepressants

Generic Name (Brand Name) Year FDA Approved *[G] denotes generic availability*	Relevant FDA Indication(s)	Available Strengths (mg)	Usual Adult Dosage Range (starting–max) (mg)
Selective serotonin reuptake inhibitor (SSRI)			
Citalopram [G] (Celexa) 1998	MDD	10, 20, 40, 10/5 mL	20–40
Escitalopram [G] (Lexapro) 2002	MDD (12+ yrs), GAD	5, 10, 20, 5/5 mL	10–20
Fluoxetine [G] (Prozac) 1987	MDD (8+ yrs), OCD (7+ yrs), panic disorder, bulimia, PMDD (as Sarafem)	10, 20, 40, 60, 20/5 mL 10, 15, 20 (Sarafem)	20–80
Fluoxetine DR [G] (Prozac Weekly) 2001	MDD maintenance	90 DR	90 Qweek
Fluvoxamine [G] Luvox brand discontinued; generic only 1994	OCD (8+ yrs)	25, 50, 100	50–300
Fluvoxamine ER [G] (Luvox CR) 2008	OCD	100, 150 ER	100–300
Paroxetine [G] (Paxil) 1992 (Pexeva) 2003 (Brisdelle) 2013	MDD, OCD, panic disorder, social anxiety, GAD, PTSD, PMDD, menopausal hot flashes (as Brisdelle)	7.5 (Brisdelle), 10, 20, 30, 40, 10/5 mL	20–60
Paroxetine CR [G] (Paxil CR) 1999	MDD, panic disorder, social anxiety, PMDD	12.5, 25, 37.5 ER	25–62.5
Sertraline [G] (Zoloft) 1991	MDD, OCD (6+ yrs), panic disorder, PTSD, PMDD, social anxiety	25, 50, 100, 150, 200, 20/mL	50–200
Serotonin norepinephrine reuptake inhibitor (SNRI)			
Desvenlafaxine [G] (Khedezla, Pristiq) 2008	MDD	25, 50, 100 ER	50–100
Duloxetine [G] (Cymbalta) 2004	MDD, GAD (7+ yrs) (also diabetic peripheral neuropathy, fibromyalgia, chronic musculoskeletal pain)	20, 30, 40, 60 DR	40–120
Levomilnacipran (Fetzima) 2013	MDD	20, 40, 80, 120 ER	20–120
Venlafaxine [G] 1993 Effexor brand discontinued; generic only	MDD	25, 37.5, 50, 75, 100	75–375
Venlafaxine ER [G] (Effexor XR) 1997	MDD, GAD, social anxiety disorder, panic disorder	37.5, 75, 150, 225 ER	75–225
Tricyclic antidepressant (TCA)			
Amitriptyline [G] Elavil brand discontinued; generic only 1961	MDD	10, 25, 50, 75, 100, 150	50–300
Clomipramine [G] (Anafranil) 1989	OCD (10+ yrs)	25, 50, 75	25–250
Desipramine [G] (Norpramin) 1964	MDD	10, 25, 50, 75, 100, 150	50–300

Generic Name (Brand Name) Year FDA Approved *[G] denotes generic availability*	Relevant FDA Indication(s)	Available Strengths (mg)	Usual Adult Dosage Range (starting–max) (mg)
Imipramine [G] Tofranil brand discontinued; generic only 1984	MDD	10, 25, 50, 75, 100, 125, 150	25–300
Nortriptyline [G] (Pamelor) 1977	MDD	10, 25, 50, 75, 10/5 mL	25–150
Monoamine oxidase inhibitor (MAOI)			
Isocarboxazid (Marplan) 1959	MDD	10	20–60
Phenelzine [G] (Nardil) 1961	MDD	15	45–90
Selegiline transdermal (EMSAM) 2006	MDD	6, 9, 12/24h patch	6/24h–12/24h
Tranylcypromine [G] (Parnate) 1961	MDD	10	30–60
Dopamine norepinephrine reuptake inhibitor			
Bupropion [G] (Wellbutrin) 1985	MDD	75, 100	200–450
Bupropion SR [G] (Wellbutrin SR) 1996	MDD, smoking cessation	100, 150, 200	150–400
Bupropion XL [G] (Wellbutrin XL, Forfivo XL) 2003	MDD, seasonal affective disorder	150, 300 (Wellbutrin XL), 450 (Forfivo XL)	150–450
Noradrenergic and specific serotonergic antidepressant (NaSSA)			
Mirtazapine [G] (Remeron) 1996	MDD	7.5, 15, 30, 45	15–45
Mirtazapine ODT [G] (Remeron SolTab) 2001	MDD	15, 30, 45	15–45
Serotonin reuptake inhibitor and 5-HT2A and 5-HT2C antagonist			
Trazodone [G] Desyrel brand discontinued; generic only 1981	MDD	50, 100, 150, 300	50–600
Serotonin reuptake inhibitor and 5-HT1A partial agonist			
Vilazodone (Viibryd) 2011	MDD	10, 20, 40	10–40
Serotonin reuptake inhibitor and 5-HT1A agonist, 5-HT1B partial agonist, and 5-HT3 & 5-HT7 antagonist			
Vortioxetine (Trintellix) 2013	MDD	5, 10, 20	10–20

BUPROPION (Wellbutrin) Fact Sheet [G]

FDA Indications:

Major depression; seasonal affective disorder; smoking cessation (as Zyban).

Off Label Uses:

ADHD; sexual dysfunction; bipolar depression.

Dosage Forms:

- **Tablets (G):** 75 mg, 100 mg.
- **SR tablets (G):** 100 mg, 150 mg, 200 mg.
- **ER tablets (G):** 150 mg, 300 mg, **Forfivo XL:** 450 mg.
- **ER tablets, hydrobromide salt formulation (Aplenzin):** 174 mg, 348 mg, 522 mg (equivalent to 150 mg, 300 mg, 450 mg, respectively).

Dosage Guidance:

- Depression (target dose 300 mg/day):
  - IR: Start 100 mg BID, ↑ to 100 mg TID after >3 days; max dose 450 mg/day, 150 mg/dose; separate doses by at least 6 hours to minimize seizure risk.
  - SR: Start 150 mg QAM, ↑ to 150 mg BID (usual target dose) as early as fourth day; max dose 400 mg/day, 200 mg/dose; separate doses by at least 8 hours to minimize seizure risk.
  - ER: Start 150 mg QAM, ↑ to 300 mg QAM as early as fourth day; max dose 450 mg QAM.

Monitoring: No routine monitoring recommended unless clinical picture warrants.

Cost: IR/SR/ER: $; Forfivo: $$$$; Aplenzin: $$$$$

Side Effects:

- Most common: Agitation, insomnia, headache, nausea, vomiting, tremor, tachycardia, dry mouth, weight loss.
- Serious but rare: Seizures; risk higher with rapid and large dose increases and in patients at risk for seizures. Risk of seizure depends on dose and formulation: IR: 300 mg/day–450 mg/day (0.4%) vs 450 mg/day–600 mg/day (4%). SR/ER: 100 mg/day–300 mg/day (0.1%) vs 400 mg/day (0.4%). Do not chew, divide, or crush SR or ER tablets as risk of seizures may be increased.

Mechanism, Pharmacokinetics, and Drug Interactions:

- Dopamine and norepinephrine receptor uptake inhibitor.
- Metabolized primarily through CYP2B6; inhibits CYP2D6; t ½: 21 hours.
- Avoid use with MAOIs.

Clinical Pearls:

- Forfivo XL offers ease of use (1 pill a day) for patients taking 450 mg/day, but it is more expensive and not yet available as generic.
- Aplenzin brand could also be a 1-pill-a-day solution (the 522 mg is equivalent to 450 mg Wellbutrin) but otherwise doesn't offer any real clinical advantage as a different salt (hydrobromide) formulation.
- Give ER dose as early in the morning as possible to minimize insomnia.
- Bupropion can cause false-positive urine test results for amphetamines.

Not-So-Fun Fact:

There have been case reports of teenagers, prisoners, and others snorting crushed tablets of bupropion (believing it to be a stimulant), with subsequent seizures.

Bottom Line:

May be particularly useful for individuals whose depression is associated with fatigue and poor concentration. Absence of sexual side effects and weight gain make this an appealing option for many depressed patients. Although not effective for anxiety disorders, it is effective for the anxiety that often accompanies depression. The seizure risk is not a concern for most patients when dosed appropriately.

DESVENLAFAXINE (Khedezla, Pristiq) Fact Sheet [G]

FDA Indications:
Major depression.

Off-Label Uses:
Fibromyalgia; vasomotor symptoms of menopause; GAD; social anxiety disorder; panic disorder; PTSD; PMDD.

Dosage Forms:
ER tablets (G): 25 mg, 50 mg, 100 mg.

Dosage Guidance:
Start 50 mg QD. Doses up to 400 mg/day have been studied, but there is no evidence of added benefit of doses >50 mg/day, only an increase in side effects.

Monitoring: Periodic blood pressure.

Cost: $$; Khedezla: $$$

Side Effects:
- Most common: Nausea, dizziness, insomnia, excessive sweating, constipation, dry mouth, somnolence, decreased appetite, anxiety, and sexual side effects.
- Serious but rare: Dose-related increases in systolic and diastolic blood pressure (as likely with Pristiq as Effexor). Monitor BP regularly, and if increases are sustained, consider reducing dose or discontinuing.

Mechanism, Pharmacokinetics, and Drug Interactions:
- Serotonin and norepinephrine reuptake inhibitor.
- Active metabolite of venlafaxine, metabolized primarily through conjugation and oxidation via CYP3A4 (minor). Minimally inhibits CYP2D6; t ½: 11 hours.
- Avoid use with MAOIs, other serotonergic medications. Not likely to cause other clinically significant interactions.

Clinical Pearls:
- Desvenlafaxine has not been shown to be any more effective than venlafaxine. Unlike venlafaxine, increasing the dose of desvenlafaxine beyond the recommended 50 mg/day likely does not improve response, but does increase side effects.
- Claims of fewer drug interactions with desvenlafaxine are likely unimportant for the majority of patients as the risk of clinically significant interactions with venlafaxine is already quite low.
- Desvenlafaxine is available in 2 forms: a succinate salt (Pristiq) and a base (Khedezla). Aside from small differences in half-life, there is no difference between these products—all efficacy studies were based on the original Pristiq studies.

Fun Fact:
Desvenlafaxine's manufacturer withdrew its application for approval in the European Union, where regulatory bodies had said that desvenlafaxine was likely less effective than venlafaxine with no advantages in terms of safety and tolerability.

Bottom Line:
For the majority of patients, there are no clear advantages to using desvenlafaxine over other agents, particularly venlafaxine XR.

DULOXETINE (Cymbalta) Fact Sheet [G]

FDA Indications:

Major depression; generalized anxiety disorder (kids ages 7+ and adults); **diabetic peripheral neuropathic pain; fibromyalgia; chronic musculoskeletal pain** (including osteoarthritis and chronic low back pain).

Off-Label Uses:

Other neuropathic or chronic pain disorders; other anxiety disorders; stress urinary incontinence.

Dosage Forms:

Capsules (delayed release) (G): 20 mg, 30 mg, 40 mg, 60 mg.

Dosage Guidance:

- Depression and GAD: Start 40 mg–60 mg/day; may be divided (20 mg or 30 mg BID) or given as a single daily dose; target dose 60 mg QD; for doses >60 mg/day, titrate in increments of 30 mg/day over 1 week to max 120 mg/day, although doses >60 mg/day not shown to be more effective.
- Fibromyalgia and chronic pain: Start 30 mg QD, increase to target 60 mg QD; max dose 60 mg/day.
- Diabetic neuropathy: Start, target, and maximum dose of 60 mg QD.

Monitoring: LFTs if suspect liver disease; periodic blood pressure.

Cost: $

Side Effects:

- Most common: Nausea, dry mouth, constipation, diarrhea, decreased appetite, vomiting, fatigue, insomnia, dizziness, agitation, sweating, headache, urinary hesitation, and sexual side effects.
- Serious but rare: Rare cases of hepatic failure (including fatalities) have been reported (too rare to require routine LFTs in all patients). Hepatitis with abdominal pain, hepatomegaly, elevated transaminases >20 times normal, with and without jaundice observed. May cause orthostatic hypotension or syncope, especially in first week of therapy and after dose increases. Urinary retention reported; hospitalization and/or catheterization were necessary in some cases.

Mechanism, Pharmacokinetics, and Drug Interactions:

- Serotonin and norepinephrine reuptake inhibitor.
- Metabolized primarily through CYP1A2 and 2D6; inhibitor of CYP2D6; t ½: 12 hours.
- Avoid use with MAOIs, other serotonergic medications. Caution with drugs metabolized by CYP2D6 (eg, paroxetine, fluoxetine, aripiprazole, iloperidone, risperidone, atomoxetine, beta blockers) as their levels may be increased. Potent inhibitors of CYP2D6 (eg, paroxetine, fluoxetine, quinidine) and CYP1A2 (eg, fluvoxamine, ciprofloxacin) may increase duloxetine levels.

Clinical Pearls:

- Since capsules are delayed release, they should be swallowed whole; do not chew or crush. Although the manufacturer does not recommend opening the capsules, their contents may be sprinkled on applesauce or in apple juice and swallowed immediately.
- Avoid in patients with a history of heavy alcohol use or chronic hepatic disease because of the possibility that duloxetine and alcohol may interact, causing hepatic injury, or the possibility that duloxetine may aggravate preexisting hepatic disease.

Fun Fact:

Duloxetine is approved in Europe for stress urinary incontinence, but the FDA refused this indication in the US because of concerns regarding liver toxicity and potential suicidal ideation.

Bottom Line:

Duloxetine has a niche for depressed patients with various comorbid pain syndromes. However, you should balance this advantage against its potentially serious hepatic side effects and pesky urinary effects.

LEVOMILNACIPRAN (Fetzima) Fact Sheet

FDA Indications:
Major depression.

Off-Label Uses:
Fibromyalgia; anxiety disorders; vasomotor symptoms of menopause; diabetic peripheral neuropathy; chronic musculoskeletal pain.

Dosage Forms:
ER capsules: 20 mg, 40 mg, 80 mg, 120 mg.

Dosage Guidance:
Start 20 mg QD; increase to 40 mg QD after 2 days, then by increments of 40 mg/day every 2 or more days to max 120 mg QD.

Monitoring: Periodic blood pressure and pulse.

Cost: $$$$

Side Effects:
- Most common: Nausea, vomiting, constipation, sweating, increased heart rate (7–9 beats/minute), erectile dysfunction, and urinary hesitation.
- Serious but rare: Urinary retention; increased blood pressure and tachycardia possible.

Mechanism, Pharmacokinetics, and Drug Interactions:
- Serotonin and norepinephrine reuptake inhibitor.
- Metabolized primarily through CYP3A4; t ½: 12 hours.
- Avoid use with MAOIs, other serotonergic medications. Use lower doses (no more than 80 mg/day) in presence of potent 3A4 inhibitors (eg, ketoconazole).

Clinical Pearls:
- Three 8-week studies showed greater efficacy than placebo at doses of 40 mg/day and greater. No head-to-head studies versus other antidepressants are available to date.
- According to the manufacturer, levomilnacipran has greater potency for norepinephrine reuptake inhibition than for serotonin reuptake inhibition.
- Noradrenergic effects may contribute to urinary hesitation or retention in about 4%–6% of patients and is dose-related.
- Nausea may be severe for many patients, especially early in treatment. Start 20 mg/day and titrate slowly to minimize as patients may develop tolerance.
- Do not cut, crush, chew, or dissolve; swallow extended release tablets whole with fluid.

Fun Fact:
Levomilnacipran is an enantiomer of milnacipran (Savella, also a Forest Pharmaceuticals drug), an SNRI approved for fibromyalgia. Milnacipran has not shown robust antidepressant efficacy and does not have that indication in the US, although it is used for depression in other countries.

Bottom Line:
Higher cost, nausea, need for titration, and urinary effects make this a second-line SNRI after venlafaxine. Use this in patients who have tried and failed other SNRIs and could benefit from greater noradrenergic effects.

MIRTAZAPINE (Remeron) Fact Sheet [G]

FDA Indications:
Major depression.

Off-Label Uses:
Panic disorder; PTSD; generalized anxiety disorder; insomnia; nausea; appetite stimulant.

Dosage Forms:
- **Tablets (G):** 7.5 mg, 15 mg, 30 mg, 45 mg.
- **Orally disintegrating tablets (G):** 15 mg, 30 mg, 45 mg.

Dosage Guidance:
Start 15 mg QHS, ↑ by 15 mg/day every 1–2 weeks. Max 45 mg/day.

Monitoring: Weight.

Cost: $

Side Effects:
- Most common: Somnolence, increased appetite, weight gain.
- Serious but rare: Agranulocytosis or severe neutropenia (with or without infection) reported very rarely.

Mechanism, Pharmacokinetics, and Drug Interactions:
- Noradrenergic (via central presynaptic alpha-2 adrenergic receptor antagonist activity) and specific serotonergic (via postsynaptic 5HT2 and 5HT3 antagonist effects) antidepressant.
- Metabolized primarily through CYP1A2, 2D6, and 3A4; t ½: 20–40 hours.
- Avoid use with MAOIs, other serotonergic agents. Caution with inducers of 1A2 or 3A4 (eg, carbamazepine), which could reduce efficacy of mirtazapine.

Clinical Pearls:
- One large meta-analysis reported that mirtazapine has a faster onset of action than other antidepressants.
- If patients experience too much sedation at initial lower dose, increase dose; mirtazapine has increased noradrenergic effect relative to antihistaminergic effect at higher doses.

Fun Fact:
Esmirtazapine, the S-enantiomer, was under development for the treatment of insomnia and hot flashes associated with menopause, but the company pulled the plug in 2010.

Bottom Line:
Mirtazapine is probably under-prescribed, likely due to concerns about weight gain and sedation. It is particularly useful in depressed patients with anxiety or insomnia, those who have had sexual side effects with other antidepressants, and those who may benefit from appetite stimulation (eg, elderly, cancer patients).

MONOAMINE OXIDASE INHIBITORS (MAOIs) Fact Sheet [G]

FDA Indications:
Major depression.

Off-Label Uses:
Treatment-resistant depression; panic disorder; social anxiety disorder.

Dosage Forms:
- Isocarboxazid, **tablets (Marplan):** 10 mg (scored).
- Phenelzine, **tablets (Nardil, G):** 15 mg.
- Tranylcypromine, **tablets (Parnate, G):** 10 mg.

Dosage Guidance:
- Isocarboxazid: Start 10 mg BID, ↑ by 10 mg/day every 2–4 days, to 40 mg/day by end of the first week (divided BID–QID). After first week, may ↑ by up to 20 mg weekly to max 60 mg/day. Use caution in patients on >40 mg/day.
- Phenelzine: Start 15 mg BID, ↑ by 15 mg/day every 2–4 days, up to 60 mg–90 mg/day divided BID.
- Tranylcypromine: Start 10 mg BID, ↑ by 10 mg/day every 2–3 weeks to maximum of 60 mg/day divided BID.

Monitoring: No routine monitoring recommended unless clinical picture warrants.

Cost: Marplan: $$$$; phenelzine: $$; tranylcypromine: $$$$

Side Effects:
- Most common: Dizziness, headache, orthostatic hypotension, dry mouth, constipation, drowsiness, tremor, sweating, peripheral edema, sexual side effects, weight gain.
- Serious but rare: Hypertensive crisis (see drug interactions).

Mechanism, Pharmacokinetics, and Drug Interactions:
- Non-selective monoamine oxidase inhibitors.
- Metabolized primarily through liver, limited data though likely through oxidative CYP450; t ½ irrelevant as irreversible inhibition effects continue for 2 weeks after discontinued.
- Avoid with other antidepressants, serotonergic agents, stimulants, sympathomimetics, dextromethorphan, disulfiram, meperidine. Do not use within 5 weeks of fluoxetine discontinuation or 2 weeks of other antidepressant discontinuation. Discontinue at least 10 days prior to elective surgery. Antihypertensives may exaggerate hypotensive effects.
- Avoid use with foods or supplements high in tyramine, tryptophan, phenylalanine, or tyrosine. Examples include aged cheese, air-dried or cured meats (eg, salami), fava or broad bean pods, tap/draft beers, Marmite concentrate, sauerkraut, soy sauce, or spoiled foods.

Clinical Pearls:
- Studies in the 1970s and 1980s showed that MAOIs were more effective than TCAs for atypical depression, characterized by overeating, oversleeping, rejection sensitivity, and mood reactivity.
- Rough dose equivalents: 20 mg of tranylcypromine = 40 mg of isocarboxazid = 45 mg phenelzine.
- When switching from an MAOI to another antidepressant, wait 2 weeks after MAOI discontinuation. This is because monoamine enzymes are irreversibly inhibited by these MAOIs, and regeneration of enzymes takes 2–3 weeks after discontinuation.

Fun Fact:
MAOIs were the first antidepressants developed, after tuberculosis patients given the antibacterial agent isoniazid (INH) were found to have an elevated mood. Isoniazid was found to be an MAOI and was developed as the first antidepressant in the late 1950s.

Bottom Line:
Not commonly used due to side effects, dietary restrictions, and drug interactions; however, MAOIs should be considered for appropriate patients who do not tolerate or respond to other antidepressants.

SELECTIVE SEROTONIN REUPTAKE INHIBITORS (SSRIs) Fact Sheet [G]

See Tables 3 and 3.1 for **medication names, FDA indication(s), off-label use, supplied as, costs, dosing, pharmacokinetics, and drug interaction information**. (Year of FDA approval can be found in Table 2.)

Monitoring: Sodium in patients at risk; ECG in patients on citalopram >40 mg/day or if cardiac disease.

Side Effects:

- Most common (SSRI with highest incidence in parentheses): Nausea (sertraline), insomnia and anxiety (fluoxetine), constipation (paroxetine), sedation (paroxetine), sexual side effects (all, but most with paroxetine), weight gain (most with paroxetine), apathy, headache.
- Serious but rare: Hyponatremia, mainly in the elderly; gastrointestinal bleeding, especially when combined with NSAIDs such as ibuprofen.
- Avoid use with MAOIs (5-week washout period with fluoxetine, 2-week washout period with all others); avoid other serotonergic agents (serotonin syndrome).
- Fluoxetine, fluvoxamine, and paroxetine are most likely to cause clinically significant P450 interactions.

Clinical Pearls:

- All SSRIs are generally equivalent in terms of efficacy. Medication selection is usually made based on side effect profile, potential for drug-drug interactions, insurance coverage, and patient preference.
- Citalopram's maximum daily dose was reduced to 40 mg/day by the FDA in August 2011 due to data suggesting increased QTc interval prolongation at doses >40 mg/day. Mean QTc interval prolongation at 60 mg/day was 18.5 msec (vs ziprasidone which has been shown to increase this interval by 20.6 msec). As of this writing, no comparable warning has been issued for escitalopram.
- Escitalopram (which is purified from the racemic mixture, citalopram) is considered the "purest" SSRI and has few, if any, drug-drug interactions.
- Fluoxetine is favored in patients who could use some activation; it is most likely to cause insomnia, anxiety, and decreased appetite.
- Fluvoxamine is used less often due to twice-daily dosing, risk for drug interactions, and fewer data for uses other than OCD even though it's likely just as effective as other SSRIs.
- Paroxetine is least favored due to side effect profile (greatest sexual side effects, weight gain, sedation, constipation) and drug interaction profile.
- Generally, higher doses of SSRIs are required for treating OCD.
- Use lower initial dose for patients with anxiety disorders, particularly panic disorder.
- SSRIs are sometimes prescribed off-label for menopausal symptoms (hot flashes), somatoform disorders, pain syndromes, migraines, and premature ejaculation.

Fun Fact:

SSRIs were the first class of psychotropic drugs discovered using rational drug design, a process that starts with a specific biological target and then creates a molecule designed to affect it.

Bottom Line:

SSRIs have become a mainstay for the treatment of patients with depression and anxiety disorders. Consider them as first-line treatment for many patients and be familiar with at least a couple of agents within the class.

TABLE 3: Selective Serotonin Reuptake Inhibitors (SSRIs)

Generic Name (Brand Name) *[G] denotes generic availability*	Relevant FDA Indication(s)	Available Strengths (mg except where noted)	Usual Dosage Range (starting–max) (mg)	Off-Label Use(s)	Cost (Cost for generic, unless otherwise specified)
Citalopram [G] (Celexa)	MDD	10, 20, 40 tabs, 10/5 mL	20 QD–40 QD Increase by 20 mg/day in 7d	OCD, PTSD, social anxiety, GAD, panic disorder, PMDD	$
Escitalopram [G] (Lexapro)	MDD (12+ yrs), GAD	5, 10, 20 tabs, 5/5 mL	10 QD–20 QD Increase by 10 mg/day in 7d	OCD, PTSD, social anxiety, panic disorder, PMDD	$ Liquid: $$
Fluoxetine [G] (Prozac, Prozac Weekly, Sarafem)	MDD (8+ yrs), OCD (7+ yrs), panic disorder, bulimia, PMDD (as Sarafem)	10, 20, 40, 60 caps/tabs; 90 DR (Prozac weekly); 20/5 mL; 10, 15, 20 tabs (Sarafem)	20 QAM–80 QAM Increase by 10 mg/day after several weeks. (Starting dose DR: 90 Qweek)	PTSD, social anxiety	$ Weekly: $$$ Sarafem: $$$$$
Fluvoxamine [G] (Luvox, Luvox CR)	OCD (8+ yrs)	25, 50, 100 IR tabs; 100, 150 ER caps	50 QHS–300 QHS Increase by 50 mg/day Qweek. (Starting dose CR: 100 QHS)	MDD, panic disorder, GAD, PTSD	$ ER: $$$
Paroxetine [G] (Brisdelle, Paxil, Paxil CR, Pexeva)	MDD, OCD, panic disorder, social anxiety, GAD, PTSD, PMDD, menopausal hot flashes (as Brisdelle)	10, 20, 30, 40 tabs; 10/5 mL; 12.5, 25, 37.5 ER; 7.5 (Brisdelle)	20 mg QHS–60 QHS CR: 25 QD–62.5 QD Increase by 10 mg/day Qweek; CR: 12.5 mg/day Qweek	Premature ejaculation	$ ER: $$ Brisdelle: $$$ Liquid, Pexeva: $$$$
Sertraline [G] (Zoloft)	MDD, OCD (6+ yrs), panic disorder, PTSD, PMDD, social anxiety	25, 50, 100, 150, 200 tabs; 20/mL	50 QD–200 QD Increase by 50 mg/day Qweek	GAD	$

TABLE 3.1: Pharmacokinetics and Drug Interactions of SSRIs

SSRI	Metabolized by (major pathways in bold)	Inhibits (potent inhibition in bold)	Elimination half-life
Citalopram	**2C19, 3A4**	2D6 (weak)	35 h
Escitalopram	**2C19, 3A4**	2D6 (weak)	27–32 h
Fluoxetine	**2D6**	**2C9/19, 2D6,** 3A4	4–6 days fluoxetine; 9 days norfluoxetine (metabolite)
Fluvoxamine	**1A2, 2D6**	**1A2, 2C9/19, 3A4**	16 h
Paroxetine	**2D6**	**2D6**	21 h
Sertraline	**2C19,** 2D6, 3A4	2D6 (weak; moderate at high dose), 3A4 (weak)	26 h

SELEGILINE TRANSDERMAL (EMSAM) Fact Sheet

FDA Indications:
Major depression.

Off-Label Uses:
Treatment-resistant depression; panic disorder; treatment-resistant anxiety disorders.

Dosage Forms:
Transdermal patch: 6 mg, 9 mg, 12 mg/24 hour patch.

Dosage Guidance:
- Start 6 mg/24 hours QD; may ↑ in increments of 3 mg/24 h every 2 weeks or more, up to max 12 mg/24 hours.
- Apply to clean, dry, intact skin to upper torso (below neck and above waist), upper thigh, or outer surface of upper arm; apply at the same time each day and rotate application sites; wash hands with soap and water after handling; avoid touching sticky side of patch.

Monitoring: No routine monitoring recommended unless clinical picture warrants.

Cost: $$$$$

Side Effects:
- Most common: Headache, insomnia, application site reaction, hypotension, diarrhea, dry mouth.
- Serious but rare: Orthostatic hypotension; caution in patients at risk (elderly, cerebrovascular disease, cardiovascular disease, hypovolemia).

Mechanism, Pharmacokinetics, and Drug Interactions:
- Non-selective MAOI.
- Metabolized primarily through CYP2B6 (also 2C9, 3A4/5) to active (N-desmethylselegiline, amphetamine, methamphetamine) and inactive metabolites; t ½: 18–25 hours.
- Avoid with other antidepressants, serotonergic agents, stimulants, sympathomimetics, dextromethorphan, disulfiram, meperidine, and carbamazepine. Do not use within 5 weeks of fluoxetine discontinuation or 2 weeks of other antidepressant discontinuation. Discontinue at least 10 days prior to elective surgery. Antihypertensives may exaggerate hypotensive effects. For doses higher than 6 mg, avoid use with foods or supplements high in tyramine, tryptophan, phenylalanine, or tyrosine.
- Wait 2 weeks after discontinuing transdermal selegiline before initiating therapy with serotonergic or any other contraindicated drug.

Clinical Pearls:
- Oral selegiline (Eldepryl) used in Parkinson's disease (≤10 mg/day) is a selective inhibitor of MAO-B, which metabolizes dopamine. When used transdermally as EMSAM, selegiline achieves higher blood levels and non-selectively inhibits both MAO-A and MAO-B. Its antidepressant effect is thought to be due to its MAO-A inhibition, which blocks the breakdown of other centrally active neurotransmitters (norepinephrine, serotonin).
- When using the 6 mg/day patch, no special diet is required. When using higher doses, a tyramine-restricted diet should be followed.
- Patch may contain conducting metal (eg, aluminum); avoid exposure of application site to external heat source, which may increase the amount of drug absorbed.

Fun Fact:
Named "EMSAM" after Emily and Samuel, the children of the CEO of Somerset Pharmaceuticals (original manufacturer).

Bottom Line:
While EMSAM is rarely used, there are some potential advantages, including compliance with patients who do not like swallowing pills; less suicide risk (harder to overdose on a patch than with pills); less likelihood of dietary interactions at 6 mg, and possibly at higher doses too; probably fewer side effects than other MAOIs, such as weight gain and sexual side effects. When MAOIs are indicated, this may be the least risky option to try.

TRAZODONE Fact Sheet [G]

FDA Indications:
Major depression.

Off-Label Uses:
Insomnia; anxiety.

Dosage Forms:
Tablets (G): 50 mg, 100 mg, 150 mg, 300 mg (scored).

Dosage Guidance:
- Depression: Start 50 mg TID; ↑ by 50 mg/day every 3–4 days to response (usually 300 mg–400 mg/day); max 600 mg/day.
- Insomnia (off-label): Start 25 mg–50 mg QHS; may ↑ by 50 mg increments up to 200 mg QHS.

Monitoring: No routine monitoring recommended unless clinical picture warrants.

Cost: $

Side Effects:
- Most common: Drowsiness, dry mouth, dizziness or lightheadedness, orthostatic hypotension, headache, blurred vision, nausea, or vomiting.
- Serious but rare: Reports of priapism (painful erection >6 hours in duration); may require surgical or pharmacologic (eg, epinephrine) intervention and may result in impotence or permanent impairment of erectile function. Orthostatic hypotension and syncope reported (less at hypnotic doses).

Mechanism, Pharmacokinetics, and Drug Interactions:
- Serotonin reuptake inhibitor, alpha-1 adrenergic receptor antagonist, and serotonin 5HT2A and 5HT2C receptor antagonist.
- Metabolized primarily through CYP3A4 to active metabolite (mCPP), which in turn is metabolized by 2D6; induces P-glycoprotein; t ½: 7–10 hours.
- Avoid use with MAOIs.

Clinical Pearls:
- If daytime drowsiness occurs, administer the majority of dosage at bedtime or ↓ dose.
- Trazodone's hypnotic effects are not due to anticholinergic nor antihistaminergic effects.
- Rarely used as antidepressant due to risk for over-sedation and orthostasis at therapeutic doses; majority of use currently is for insomnia.

Fun Fact:
As a consequence of the production of mCPP as a metabolite, patients taking trazodone may test positive on urine tests for the presence of MDMA (ecstasy).

Bottom Line:
Fewer sexual side effects and less weight gain compared to other serotonergic antidepressants make this drug appealing for depression. But significant daytime somnolence and dizziness, as well as questionable efficacy for depression at doses ≤375 mg/day, limit the utility of trazodone in depression. Trazodone continues to be a go-to drug for many patients with insomnia.

TRICYCLIC ANTIDEPRESSANTS (TCAs) Fact Sheet [G]

FDA Indications:

Major depression, obsessive compulsive disorder (OCD).

Off-Label Uses:

Headache; neuropathic pain; fibromyalgia; anxiety disorders; insomnia.

Dosage Forms:

- **Amitriptyline tablets (G):** 10 mg, 25 mg, 50 mg, 75 mg, 100 mg, 150 mg.
- **Clomipramine capsules (Anafranil, G):** 25 mg, 50 mg, 75 mg.
- **Desipramine tablets (Norpramin, G):** 10 mg, 25 mg, 50 mg, 75 mg, 100 mg, 150 mg.
- **Imipramine tablets and capsules (G):** 10 mg, 25 mg, 50 mg, 75 mg, 100 mg, 125 mg, 150 mg.
- **Nortriptyline capsules (Pamelor, G):** 10 mg, 25 mg, 50 mg, 75 mg, and 10 mg/5 mL oral solution.

Dosage Guidance:

- Amitriptyline or imipramine: Start 25 mg–50 mg QHS and ↑ by 25 mg–50 mg/day intervals every 2–3 days to target dose 150 mg–200 mg/day; max 300 mg/day.
- Clomipramine: Start 25 mg QHS and ↑ by 25 mg/day every 4–7 days to target dose 150 mg–250 mg/day; max 250 mg/day.
- Desipramine: Start 25 mg–50 mg QHS and ↑ by 25 mg–50 mg/day intervals every 2–3 days to target dose 150 mg–200 mg/day; max 300 mg/day.
- Nortriptyline: Start 25 mg–50 mg QHS and ↑ by 25 mg–50 mg/day intervals every 2–3 days to target dose 50 mg–150 mg/day; max 150 mg/day.

Monitoring: ECG if history of cardiac disease.

Cost: Amitriptyline: $; clomipramine: $$$; desipramine: $$; imipramine: $; nortriptyline: $

Side Effects:

- Most common: Sedation, dry mouth, constipation, weight gain, sexual side effects, urinary hesitation, blurred vision.
- Serious but rare: Seizure; cardiac effects including orthostasis, arrhythmias, QT prolongation, AV block.

Mechanism, Pharmacokinetics, and Drug Interactions:

- Serotonin and norepinephrine reuptake inhibitors.
- Metabolized primarily through liver (limited data, though likely through oxidative CYP2D6 primarily); t ½: 18–44 hours.
- Avoid use with other serotonergic antidepressants or agents with hypotensive or anticholinergic effects.

Clinical Pearls:

- Using divided doses (BID to TID) may help with tolerability during initiation and titration; but can convert to QHS dosing to minimize daytime sedation.
- Tertiary amines amitriptyline and imipramine are metabolized to secondary amines nortriptyline and desipramine, respectively. Secondary amines are generally better tolerated.
- Serum level monitoring established for some TCAs (amitriptyline + nortriptyline: 120–250 ng/mL; desipramine: >115–250 ng/mL; nortriptyline: 50–150 ng/mL).
- Overdose toxicity with potentially serious cardiac effects or fatality with as little as 10-day supply.

Fun Fact:

Imipramine was the first antidepressant approved in the US, developed by tweaking the molecular structure of the antipsychotic Thorazine. It didn't work for psychosis, but was the first wonder drug for depression and anxiety.

Bottom Line:

Not commonly used due to side effects and overdose toxicity risk; however, TCAs should be considered for appropriate patients who do not respond to other antidepressants.

VENLAFAXINE (Effexor XR) Fact Sheet [G]

FDA Indications:

Major depression, social anxiety disorder, GAD, panic disorder.

Off-Label Uses:

PTSD; PMDD; vasomotor symptoms of menopause; diabetic peripheral neuropathy.

Dosage Forms:

- **Tablets (G):** 25 mg, 37.5 mg, 50 mg, 75 mg, 100 mg (scored).
- **ER tablets (G):** 37.5 mg, 75 mg, 150 mg, 225 mg.

Dosage Guidance:

- Depression:
  Start 75 mg/day in 2–3 divided doses or as XR once daily; ↑ dose by 75 mg/day at intervals of 4 or more days; max 375 mg/day (divided TID) or 225 mg/day XR given once daily. IR may be switched to nearest equivalent daily dose of XR QD.
- Anxiety:
  XR: Start 75 mg QD, ↑ by 75 mg/day at weekly intervals; max 225 mg/day; for panic disorder, to minimize exacerbation of panic, start 37.5 mg QD, ↑ to 75 mg QD after 1 week then by 75 mg/day at weekly intervals; max 225 mg/day.

Monitoring: Periodic blood pressure.

Cost: IR: $; ER: $$

Side Effects:

- Most common: Anorexia, constipation, dizziness, dry mouth, nausea, nervousness, somnolence, sweating, sexual side effects, headache, insomnia.
- Serious but rare: Sustained, dose-related hypertension reported. May cause hyponatremia or SIADH; use with caution in patients who are volume-depleted, elderly, or taking diuretics.

Mechanism, Pharmacokinetics, and Drug Interactions:

- Serotonin and norepinephrine reuptake inhibitor.
- Metabolized primarily through CYP2D6 to O-desmethylvenlafaxine (ODV), major active metabolite (an SNRI, marketed as Pristiq) and also by CYP3A4; t ½: 5 hours (11 hours for ODV).
- Avoid use with MAOIs, other serotonergic agents. Caution with CYP2D6 or 3A4 inhibitors, which may increase venlafaxine levels. Inhibits CYP2D6.

Clinical Pearls:

- For patients with nausea, start at lower dose, titrate more slowly, and give with food.
- May cause false-positive PCP in urine drug screen.
- Increase in blood pressure much more likely in doses >225 mg/day.
- Significant discontinuation syndrome, even with XR formulation.
- Theoretically functions as an SSRI in low doses (75 mg/day) and as an SNRI in moderate doses (150 mg–225 mg/day), and affects all monoamines in high doses (>225 mg/day).
- No additional benefit seen with doses >225 mg/day in moderately depressed outpatients, but patients with more severe depression may respond to higher doses (350 mg/day).

Fun Fact:

Venlafaxine is structurally related to the atypical opioid analgesic tramadol (Ultram) (itself a serotonergic agent), but not to any other antidepressant drugs.

Bottom Line:

Venlafaxine is probably somewhat more effective than SSRIs for depression, with a number needed to treat (NNT) of around 15, but its side effect disadvantages relegate it to second-line use.

VILAZODONE (Viibryd) Fact Sheet

FDA Indications:
Major depression.

Off-Label Uses:
OCD; other anxiety disorders.

Dosage Forms:
Tablets: 10 mg, 20 mg, 40 mg.

Dosage Guidance:
- Start 10 mg QD for 7 days; ↑ to 20 mg QD for 7 days, then to recommended dose of 20 mg–40 mg QD (with food). Purpose of dose titration is to minimize GI effects.
- Must take with food, otherwise serum levels are reduced by up to 50%.

Monitoring: No routine monitoring recommended unless clinical picture warrants.

Cost: $$$$

Side Effects:
- Most common: Diarrhea, nausea, vomiting, dry mouth, insomnia, dizziness.
- Serious but rare: Possible hyponatremia or SIADH; use with caution in patients who are volume-depleted, elderly, or taking diuretics.

Mechanism, Pharmacokinetics, and Drug Interactions:
- SSRI plus 5-HT1A partial agonist (buspirone is also 5-HT1A partial agonist).
- Metabolized primarily through CYP3A4; t ½: 25 hours.
- Avoid use with MAOIs, other serotonergic agents. More P450 drug interactions possible with vilazodone than some other SSRIs: Use with 3A4 inhibitors or inducers may require dose adjustment.

Clinical Pearl:
Sometimes marketed as having no or few sexual side effects, but FDA officials wrote an article for *Journal of Clinical Psychiatry* clarifying that studies do not support this claim.

Fun Guess:
The brand name "Viibryd" likely has two origins. First, it rhymes with "hybrid," and the mechanism of action is a hybrid of SSRI and 5-HT1A partial agonism. Second, the word calls to mind "virile," which could be a subliminal suggestion that it does not worsen sexual functioning.

Bottom Line:
Vilazodone appears to be another SSRI (with a little buspirone thrown in). We do not yet know if it has any side effect advantages over other SSRIs. Disadvantages include the slow titration schedule, the need to take it with food in order to achieve a therapeutic blood level, and the many drug interactions. Until further notice, vilazodone should remain a second-line antidepressant.

VORTIOXETINE (Trintellix) Fact Sheet

FDA Indications:
Major depression.

Off-Label Uses:
Generalized anxiety disorder; other anxiety disorders.

Dosage Forms:
Tablets: 5 mg, 10 mg, 15 mg, 20 mg.

Dosage Guidance:
Start 10 mg QD; ↑ to 20 mg QD as tolerated. Consider 5 mg/day for those unable to tolerate higher doses.

Monitoring: No routine monitoring recommended unless clinical picture warrants.

Cost: $$$$

Side Effects:
- Most common: Nausea, constipation, vomiting, sexual side effects, dry mouth, headache.
- Serious but rare: Serotonergic antidepressants have been rarely associated with bruising or bleeding.

Mechanism, Pharmacokinetics, and Drug Interactions:
- Multi-modal antidepressant.
- Metabolized primarily through CYP2D6 and, to a lesser extent, via 3A4/5, 2C9/19, 2A6, 2C8, and 2B6; t ½: 66 hours.
- Avoid use with MAOIs, other serotonergic medications. Use lower doses in presence of potent 2D6 inhibitors.

Clinical Pearls:
- Vortioxetine is a "multimodal" antidepressant or a "serotonin modulator and stimulator." This means it has effects on several receptor sites. Like SSRIs, it is a serotonin reuptake inhibitor, but it also is an agonist at 5-HT1A receptors, a partial agonist at 5-HT1B receptors, and an antagonist at 5-HT3A, 5-HT1D, and 5-HT7 receptors.
- Some data imply a pro-cognitive effect, but at this point it isn't clear if this is a nonspecific byproduct of the drug's antidepressant effects, or a specific advantage of vortioxetine. The studies needed to sort this out have not yet been done.
- Negative findings in some studies were attributed to dose being too low (5–10 mg/day). Higher-dose studies showed vortioxetine to be as effective as both duloxetine and agomelatine, an antidepressant approved in Europe.

Fun Fact:
The original brand name of vortioxetine, Brintellix, was apparently crafted to subliminally suggest that the drug helps cognition ("**br**ing **intelli**gence"). It was changed to Trintellix in 2016 because of reports of dispensing errors between Brintellix and Brilinta, the antiplatelet medication ticagrelor.

Bottom Line:
More experience will give us a better understanding of this drug's place in therapy and if it really is different than other serotonergic antidepressants. Until then, consider it a second-line agent due to its high cost and limited track record.

Antipsychotics

GENERAL PRESCRIBING TIPS

Which antipsychotic should you choose? That's probably the most difficult question to answer in psychiatry. There are dozens of options and approved indications. Here are some of the factors you should weigh as you decide which antipsychotic to prescribe for a given patient:

- Efficacy
- Side effects
- Cost

Efficacy

While there's some debate about this, most experts consider clozapine to be the only antipsychotic that is clearly more effective than the others. That's wonderful, except that clozapine also happens to be the drug with one of the worst side effect profiles in psychiatry. Weight gain is the most prominent: You can expect half of all patients who take clozapine to have a 20% or more weight gain over time (Umbricht DS et al, *J Clin Psychiatry* 1994;55(suppl B):157–160). When you consider its other major side effects, like sedation, drooling, and life-threatening neutropenia, not to mention the necessity of monthly blood draws, it's no wonder that clozapine is used pretty rarely. Nonetheless, it's incredibly helpful for certain treatment-resistant patients.

Next on the list of drugs that might be more effective than others is olanzapine, another side effect overachiever. It doesn't cause as much weight gain as clozapine, but it's close. In the CATIE trial, 30% of patients gained at least 7% of their initial weight.

Beyond this, there's no consensus that any of the other SGAs differ in efficacy, at least for core symptoms of psychosis. It's possible that SGAs have a broader spectrum of efficacy, given that many are approved for various mood syndromes as well as psychosis. Some people believe that SGAs are more effective than FGAs for negative symptoms. This is probably an artifact of the fact that FGAs are more likely to cause side effects, like extrapyramidal symptoms (EPS), which can mimic negative symptoms. As more SGAs go generic, it is becoming more reasonable to choose them over FGAs for most patients.

Side Effects

SGAs are less likely to cause EPS and tardive dyskinesia than FGAs. Nonetheless, SGAs have plenty of side effects (see Table 6 for a side-by-side comparison), and here are some of the highlights:

- *Weight gain/hyperlipidemia/diabetes.* Clozapine is the worst, followed by Zyprexa, Seroquel, and Risperdal/Invega, in roughly descending order. All of the other SGAs are close to weight-neutral in adults, but we're less confident about this in kids, who tend to balloon up with many supposedly weight-neutral antipsychotics, including Abilify.
- *Sedation.* Clozapine, Zyprexa, and Seroquel tend to be the most sedating, though it's important to note that sedation isn't always bad. Patients who are revved up in a manic psychosis might do particularly well on a sedating antipsychotic—but you might want to switch to an alternative for long-term treatment.
- *Cardiac issues.* Here we are talking about ECG changes, rather than the more indirect cardiac effect of hyperlipidemia. Geodon is the most infamous example, and it does increase the QT interval, which in turn can theoretically cause serious arrhythmias. In practice, however, the actual risk is slight, with a 0.06% rate of clinically relevant QT prolongation. Several other antipsychotics can cause QT prolongation, including thioridazine (Mellaril), iloperidone (Fanapt), and to a lesser extent quetiapine (Seroquel).
- *EPS.* Among the FGAs, Haldol and Prolixin cause the most EPS, while risperidone is the SGA with the highest EPS risk.
- *Akathisia.* Aripiprazole (Abilify) and brexpiprazole (Rexulti) are the SGAs most likely to cause akathisia.

Cost

As of this writing, the following atypicals are available as generics, rendering them relatively inexpensive: aripiprazole, clozapine, olanzapine, paliperidone, quetiapine, risperidone, and ziprasidone.

On the other hand, the following antipsychotics are brand-name only and are often ridiculously expensive (up to, or even over, $1,000 per month): asenapine (Saphris), brexpiprazole (Rexulti), cariprazine (Vraylar), iloperidone (Fanapt), and lurasidone (Latuda).

Class Warnings

All of the atypical antipsychotics carry the same FDA class warnings. Rather than repeating all of these concerns on each fact sheet, we will mention the warnings here:

- In 2003, the FDA required all manufacturers of atypical antipsychotics to revise their package labeling to reflect the potential risks for weight gain, hyperglycemia, new-onset or worsening diabetes, and hyperlipidemias. While this has become a class warning, it's clear that there are a handful of really bad actors here: Clozapine and olanzapine are the worst, quetiapine and risperidone relatively less so.
- Patient-specific factors may also play a role. In general, the incidence and severity of weight gain and metabolic effects appear to be greater in the pediatric population.

A 2004 consensus statement from the American Psychiatric Association and American Diabetes Association recommends the following monitoring protocol for patients on atypical agents. These are the minimal recommendations for monitoring; obviously, more frequent monitoring—for example, in individuals with elevated triglycerides or blood sugar—may be more appropriate for your patients.

TABLE 4: APA/ADA Monitoring Protocol for Patients on SGAs

	Baseline	4 Weeks	8 Weeks	12 Weeks	Quarterly	Annually	Every 5 Years
Personal/Family History	X					X	
Weight (BMI)	X	X	X	X	X		
Waist Circumference	X					X	
Blood Pressure	X			X		X	
Fasting Plasma Glucose	X			X		X	
Fasting Lipid Profile	X			X			X

Republished with permission of The American Diabetes Association, from *Diabetes Care*, 27(2):2004.
Permission conveyed through Copyright Clearance Center, Inc.

- A black box warning for all agents in this class suggests a substantially **higher mortality rate in geriatric patients with dementia-related psychosis** receiving atypical antipsychotics (4.5%) compared with those receiving placebo (2.6%). Although most fatalities resulted from cardiac-related events (eg, heart failure, sudden death) or infections (mostly pneumonia) as opposed to a clearly direct effect of medication, atypical antipsychotics are *not* approved for the treatment of dementia-related psychosis, and such use should be avoided or minimized when possible.
- **Adverse cerebrovascular events** (eg, stroke, TIA), sometimes fatal, have been reported in geriatric patients (73–97 years of age) with dementia-related psychosis. The FDA has issued a black box warning on atypical antipsychotics to reflect this risk; several studies have shown that cerebrovascular event risk is elevated with typical antipsychotics, as well.

Other warnings that should be considered for all antipsychotic agents (atypicals as well as typical agents) include the following:

- **Neuroleptic malignant syndrome (NMS),** a potentially fatal syndrome characterized by fever, severe muscle rigidity, and autonomic instability, has been reported in patients receiving antipsychotic agents. Treatment requires immediate discontinuation of the drug and intensive symptomatic treatment in a hospital setting.
- **Tardive dyskinesia (TD),** a syndrome of potentially irreversible, involuntary dyskinetic movements, has been reported. TD is more common with FGAs than with atypical agents.

Extrapyramidal and withdrawal symptoms in newborns have been reported with maternal use of typical antipsychotics during the third trimester of pregnancy. Symptoms in the newborn may include agitation, feeding disorder, hypertonia or hypotonia, respiratory distress, and somnolence. These effects vary in severity and may be self-limiting (subsiding within hours or days) or, in rare cases, require hospitalization.

TABLE 5: Typical Antipsychotics

Generic Name (Brand Name) Year FDA Approved *[G] denotes generic availability*	Relevant FDA Indication(s)	Available Strengths (mg)	Dosage Equivalents	Usual Dosage Range (starting–max) (mg)	EPS and Akathisia	Anticholinergic	Relative Sedation and Orthostasis	Notes
Chlorpromazine [G] (Thorazine[1]) 1957	Psychosis, mania, nausea/vomiting	10, 25, 50, 100, 200; IM: 25 mg/mL	100	50–600	Low	Moderate	High	Injectable available; photosensitivity
Fluphenazine [G] (Prolixin[1], Prolixin Decanoate[1]) 1960	Psychosis	1, 2.5, 5, 10	2	2–20	Very high	Low	Low	Oral solution; injectables (short and LAI) available
Haloperidol [G] (Haldol, Haldol Decanoate) 1967	Psychosis, Tourette's disorder	0.5, 1, 2, 5, 10, 20	2	2–20	Very high	Low	Low	Oral solution; injectables (short and LAI) available
Loxapine [G] (Adasuve, Loxitane[1]) 1975	Schizophrenia	5, 10, 25, 50	10	20–100	High	Low	Moderate	10 mg oral inhalation powder available as Adasuve since 2012; available only in enrolled health care facilities
Molindone [G] (Moban[1]) 1974	Schizophrenia	5, 10, 25	10	50–100	High	Low	Moderate	Less weight gain than others
Perphenazine [G] (Trilafon[1]) 1957	Schizophrenia, severe nausea/vomiting	2, 4, 8, 16	8	8–64	High	Low	Low	Mid-potency agent studied and compared to atypicals in CATIE (see fact sheet)
Thioridazine [G] (Mellaril[1]) 1962	Schizophrenia	10, 25, 50, 100	100	50–600	Low	High	High	QT prolongation; irreversible retinal pigmentation at >800 mg/day
Thiothixene [G] (Navane) 1967	Schizophrenia	1, 2, 5, 10, 20	4	6–40	High	Low	Low	High-potency agent
Trifluoperazine [G] (Stelazine[1]) 1959	Schizophrenia, non-psychotic anxiety	1, 2, 5, 10	5	4–40	High	Low	Low	High-potency agent

[1]Brand discontinued; no longer available as brand

TABLE 6: Atypical Antipsychotics

Generic Name (Brand Name) Year FDA Approved *[G] denotes generic availability*	Relevant FDA Indication(s) (pediatric ages specified where relevant)	Available Strengths (mg)	Usual Dosage Range (starting–max) (mg)[1]	Weight Gain and Metabolic Effects	EPS and Akathisia	QT Prolongation	Notes
Aripiprazole [G] (Abilify, Abilify Discmelt) 2002	Schizophrenia (13+) Bipolar mania, monotherapy and adjunctive (10+) Bipolar maintenance, monotherapy and adjunctive Depression adjunct Irritability in autism (6–17) Tourette's disorder (6–18) Agitation in schizophrenia or bipolar (IM only) Acute schizophrenia relapse (LAI Maintena only)	Tablet: 2, 5, 10, 15, 20, 30 ODT: 10, 15 Liquid: 1 mg/mL LAI: Maintena (see fact sheet)	10–30 QD	Low	High (mainly akathisia)	Low	Probably most "activating"
Asenapine (Saphris) 2009	Schizophrenia Bipolar mania, monotherapy and adjunctive (10+)	Tablet: 2.5, 5, 10 (sublingual only)	5–10 BID	Moderate	Moderate	Low	Avoid food or drink for 10 minutes after taking; sedating
Brexpiprazole (Rexulti) 2015	Schizophrenia Depression adjunct	Tablet: 0.25, 0.5, 1, 2, 3, 4	1–4 QD	Moderate	High (mainly akathisia)	Low	Newer agent with limited data; weight gain and akathisia most common adverse effects
Cariprazine (Vraylar) 2015	Schizophrenia Bipolar mania and mixed episodes	Capsule: 1.5, 3, 4.5, 6	1.5–6 QD	Moderate	Moderate	Low	Newest agent with limited data; possible negative symptom efficacy
Clozapine [G] (Clozaril, FazaClo, Versacloz) 1989 Generic not available for oral suspension	Treatment-resistant schizophrenia Recurrent suicidal behavior in schizophrenia or schizoaffective disorders	Tablet: 25, 50, 100, 200 ODT: 12.5, 25, 100, 150, 200 Oral suspension: 50 mg/mL	12.5–450 BID	High	Low	Low	Probably most effective AP
Iloperidone (Fanapt) 2009	Schizophrenia	Tablet: 1, 2, 4, 6, 8, 10, 12	2–12 BID	Moderate	Low	Moderate/high	Orthostatic dizziness; must be titrated
Lurasidone (Latuda) 2010	Schizophrenia, bipolar depression	Tablet: 20, 40, 60, 80, 120	40–160 QD	Low/moderate	Moderate	Low	Sedating; must take with food

ODT = orally disintegrating tablet, LAI = long-acting injectable ER, XR = extended release

[1]For schizophrenia indication

Generic Name (Brand Name) Year FDA Approved *[G] denotes generic availability*	Relevant FDA Indication(s) (pediatric ages specified where relevant)	Available Strengths (mg)	Usual Dosage Range (starting–max) (mg)[1]	Weight Gain and Metabolic Effects	EPS and Akathisia	QT Prolongation	Notes
Olanzapine [G] (Zyprexa, Zyprexa Zydis) 1996 Generic not available for LAI	Schizophrenia (13+) Bipolar mania, monotherapy and adjunctive (13+) Bipolar maintenance, monotherapy Agitation in schizophrenia or bipolar (IM only)	Tablet: 2.5, 5, 7.5, 10, 15, 20 ODT: 5, 10, 15, 20 IM injection: 10 mg/vial LAI: Relprevv (see fact sheet)	10–20 QD	High	Low/moderate	Low	Greatest weight gain
Paliperidone [G] (Invega) 2006 Generic not available for LAI	Schizophrenia (12+) Schizoaffective disorder	ER tablet: 1.5, 3, 6, 9 LAI: Sustenna and Trinza (see fact sheet)	6–12 QD	Moderate	High	Moderate	Good for those with hepatic impairment; increases prolactin
Pimavanserin (Nuplazid) 2016	Parkinson's disease psychosis	Tablet: 17	34 QD	Low	Low	Low	No data in schizophrenia
Quetiapine [G] (Seroquel) 1997 (Seroquel XR) 2007	Schizophrenia (13+) Bipolar mania, monotherapy and adjunctive (10+) Bipolar disorder maintenance Bipolar depression Depression adjunct (approved in ER form)	Tablet: 25, 50, 100, 200, 300, 400 ER tablet: 50, 150, 200, 300, 400	50–800 QD; daily; divided BID to TID 300–800 QHS for XR	Moderate	Low	Moderate	Sedating
Risperidone [G] (Risperdal, Risperdal M-Tab) 1993 Generic not available for LAI	Schizophrenia (13+) Bipolar mania, monotherapy and adjunctive (10+) Irritability in autism (ages 5–16)	Liquid: 1 mg/mL Tablet: 0.25, 0.5, 1, 2, 3, 4 ODT: 0.25, 0.5, 1, 2, 3, 4 LAI: Consta (see fact sheet)	2–6 divided QD to BID	Moderate	High	Low	Increases prolactin
Ziprasidone [G] (Geodon) 2001 Generic not available for IM	Schizophrenia Bipolar mania, monotherapy Bipolar maintenance adjunctive Agitation in schizophrenia (IM injection)	Capsule: 20, 40, 60, 80 IM injection: 20 mg/mL	20–80 BID	Low	Low	High	Take with food

ODT = orally disintegrating tablet, LAI = long-acting injectable ER, XR = extended release

[1]For schizophrenia indication

Antipsychotics

ARIPIPRAZOLE (Abilify) Fact Sheet [G]

FDA Indications:

Schizophrenia (adults, adolescents 13–17 years); **bipolar disorder,** acute treatment of manic and mixed episodes (adults, children 10–17 years); bipolar disorder, maintenance treatment (adults); **major depression,** as adjunct (adults); **irritability in autism** (children 6–17 years); **Tourette's disorder** (children 6–18 years).

Off-Label Uses:

Bipolar depression; behavioral disturbances.

Dosage Forms:

- **Tablets (G):** 2 mg, 5 mg, 10 mg, 15 mg, 20 mg, 30 mg.
- **Orally disintegrating tablets (G):** 10 mg, 15 mg.
- **Oral liquid (G):** 1 mg/mL.
- **IM depot:** Abilify Maintena: 300 mg and 400 mg; Aristada: 441 mg, 662 mg, 882 mg, 1064 mg (see LAI table).
- **Tablet with sensor** (Abilify MyCite): 2 mg, 5 mg, 10 mg, 15 mg, 20 mg, 30 mg.

Dosage Guidance:

- Schizophrenia and bipolar disorder: Adults: Start and target dose 10 mg–15 mg/day; max 30 mg/day. Kids: Start 2 mg/day, increase on 3rd day to 5 mg/day; may increase further by 5 mg/day increments weekly to target dose 10 mg/day, max 30 mg/day.
- Irritability in autism (peds): Start 2 mg/day, increase up to 5 mg/day in weekly increments to target dose 5–10 mg/day, max 15 mg/day.
- Depression: Start 2 mg–5 mg/day, ↑ to usual dose 5 mg–10 mg/day, as adjunct. Titrate gradually to prevent agitation/akathisia (max 15 mg/day).
- Tourette's: Start 2 mg/day, ↑ to target 5 mg/day, max 10 mg/day (<50 kg); 10 mg/day, max 20 mg/day (>50 kg).
- Depot: After oral dose tolerated, start Abilify Maintena 400 mg/4 weeks (continue oral aripiprazole for first 14 days), target dose 300 mg–400 mg/4 weeks. For Aristada: Start 441 mg, 662 mg, or 882 mg monthly—corresponds to 300 mg, 450 mg, and 600 mg of aripiprazole, respectively. Or, start 882 mg dose every 6 weeks or 1064 mg dose every 2 months. For all Aristada regimens, continue oral aripiprazole for first 21 days.
- Liquid dosing: Oral solution equivalent to tablet dose up to 25 mg; for 30 mg tablets, give 25 mg oral solution.
- Orally disintegrating tablet: Same as regular tablet dosing.

Monitoring: Fasting glucose, lipids.

Cost: $$; ODT, liquid: $$$$

Side Effects:

- Most common: Akathisia, anxiety, insomnia, sedation, tremors.
- Serious but rare: Rare reports of reversible pathologic gambling and other impulse control problems (eating, spending, sexual).

Mechanism, Pharmacokinetics, and Drug Interactions:

- Dopamine D2 and serotonin 5HT1A receptor partial agonist and serotonin 5HT2A receptor antagonist.
- Metabolized by CYP450 2D6 and 3A4; t ½: 3 to 6 days.
- Use ½ usual dose in presence of 2D6 or 3A4 inhibitors or in known 2D6 poor metabolizers; ¼ dose if both 2D6 inhibitor/poor metabolizer and 3A4 inhibitors; double dose if also using 3A4 inducer.

Clinical Pearl:

- Some prescribers use low-dose aripiprazole to counteract antipsychotic-induced prolactinemia, given its partial agonist properties.
- In November 2017 FDA approved Abilify MyCite, which is aripiprazole with an embedded ingestible sensor to track adherence.

Fun Fact:

After aripiprazole's generic launch, Otsuka followed up with brexpiprazole (see fact sheet), another dopamine partial agonist, approved for schizophrenia and depression (as adjunct) and in clinical trials for ADHD.

Bottom Line:

Good choice for minimizing risk of weight gain and metabolic side effects, but beware of akathisia. Large number of indications and reports of success at a variety of doses make it difficult to predict dosing for individual patients.

ASENAPINE (Saphris) Fact Sheet

FDA Indications:

Schizophrenia; bipolar disorder, acute and maintenance treatment of manic or mixed episodes (adults, children 10–17 years).

Off-Label Uses:

Bipolar maintenance; bipolar depression; behavioral disturbances; impulse control disorders.

Dosage Forms:

SL tablets: 2.5 mg, 5 mg, 10 mg. (Must be taken sublingually because if swallowed, too much medication is metabolized by the liver during first-pass metabolism.)

Dosage Guidance:

- Schizophrenia: Start 5 mg BID, and increase as needed up to 10 mg BID.
- Bipolar (adults): Same dosing as schizophrenia.
- Bipolar (peds): Start 2.5 mg BID, increase as needed up to 10 mg BID.
- Do not swallow tablets. Avoid food or drink for 10 minutes after taking (they significantly reduce absorption and bioavailability).

Monitoring: Fasting glucose, lipids.

Cost: $$$$$

Side Effects:

- Most common: Akathisia (seems to be dose-related), oral hypoesthesia (numbing of the tongue or decreased oral sensitivity), somnolence, dizziness, extrapyramidal symptoms, weight gain.
- Serious but rare: Hypersensitivity reactions including anaphylaxis, angioedema, low blood pressure, rapid heart rate, swollen tongue, difficulty breathing, wheezing, or rash; orthostatic hypotension and syncope, particularly early in treatment (FDA warning, 9/2011).

Mechanism, Pharmacokinetics, and Drug Interactions:

- Dopamine D2 and serotonin 5HT2A receptor antagonist.
- Metabolized by glucuronidation and CYP1A2; t ½: 24 hours. Inhibitor of 2D6; may double paroxetine levels. Smoking may induce metabolism and may lower levels of asenapine via 1A2 induction; adjust dosing. CYP1A2 inhibitors (eg, fluvoxamine) may increase levels of asenapine; adjust dose.
- Caution with antihypertensive agents and other drugs that can cause additive hypotension or bradycardia.

Clinical Pearls:

- Has a receptor-binding profile similar to clozapine, although asenapine has very little anticholinergic activity.
- Weight gain seems to be a problem in many patients.
- Contraindicated in patients with severe hepatic impairment due to 7-fold higher levels.
- Most useful for patients who don't like swallowing pills.

Fun Fact:

Black cherry flavor developed after patients complained about original tablets.

Bottom Line:

Since there are no clear advantages over other atypical antipsychotics, the only reason to prescribe Saphris is if your patient can't or doesn't want to swallow a pill. Mouth numbness, sedation, dizziness, akathisia, weight gain, and potential for allergic reaction are significant liabilities. Not recommended for first-line use.

BREXPIPRAZOLE (Rexulti) Fact Sheet

FDA Indications:
Schizophrenia; depression adjunct.

Off-Label Uses:
Too new to tell.

Dosage Forms:
Tablets: 0.25 mg, 0.5 mg, 1 mg, 2 mg, 3 mg, 4 mg.

Dosage Guidance:
- Schizophrenia: Start 1 mg/day on days 1–4; ↑ to 2 mg/day on days 5–7; then up to max 4 mg/day based on patient response. Usual dose 2 mg–4 mg/day.
- Depression adjunct: Start 0.5 mg–1 mg/day, ↑ at weekly intervals up to target 2 mg/day, max 3 mg/day.

Monitoring: Fasting glucose, lipids.

Cost: $$$$$

Side Effects:
- Most common: Weight gain, akathisia, somnolence.
- Serious but rare: See class warnings in chapter introduction.

Mechanism, Pharmacokinetics, and Drug Interactions:
- Dopamine D2 and serotonin 5HT1A receptor partial agonist and serotonin 5HT2A receptor antagonist.
- Metabolized by CYP2D6 and 3A4; t ½: 91 hours.
- Use ½ usual dose in presence of 2D6 or 3A4 inhibitors or in known 2D6 poor metabolizers; ¼ dose if both 2D6 inhibitor/poor metabolizer and 3A4 inhibitors; double dose if also using 3A4 inducer.

Clinical Pearls:
- As the name suggests, brexpiprazole is chemically and structurally related to its manufacturer's previous blockbuster aripiprazole (Abilify).
- Although the FDA-approved target dose for schizophrenia is 2–4 mg/day, 2 mg/day was no better than placebo in 1 of 2 preclinical registration studies.
- Once-a-day dosing with no regard to meals makes this an easy-to-use option.

Fun Fact:
Plan on seeing more trial results with Rexulti in the future, including those in patients with attention-deficit/hyperactivity disorder, posttraumatic stress disorder, and agitation associated with Alzheimer's dementia.

Bottom Line:
Rexulti may just be a newer spin on Abilify, which is now available as generic. More trial data, especially long-term and compared to other antipsychotic agents, will indicate whether this is a different chemical entity that warrants a higher price tag. Until then, stick to the cheaper, generic aripiprazole.

CARIPRAZINE (Vraylar) Fact Sheet

FDA Indications:

Schizophrenia; acute treatment of **bipolar disorder (manic or mixed episodes).**

Off-Label Uses:

Negative symptoms of schizophrenia; major depression; bipolar depression.

Dosage Forms:

Capsules: 1.5 mg, 3 mg, 4.5 mg, 6 mg.

Dosage Guidance:

Schizophrenia and bipolar disorder: Start 1.5 mg/day, increase to 3 mg/day as early as 2nd day. Adjust by 1.5 mg–3 mg/day increments to usual dose 1.5 mg–6 mg/day in schizophrenia and 3 mg–6 mg/day in bipolar disorder.

Monitoring: Fasting glucose, lipids.

Cost: $$$$$

Side Effects:

- Most common: EPS, akathisia, weight gain, sedation.
- Serious but rare: See class warnings in chapter introduction.

Mechanism, Pharmacokinetics, and Drug Interactions:

- Dopamine D2 and D3 and serotonin 5HT1A receptor partial agonist; serotonin 5HT2A receptor antagonist.
- Metabolized primarily by CYP3A4; t ½: 2–4 days for cariprazine (1–3 weeks for active metabolites).
- Caution with CYP3A4 inhibitors; 50% dose reduction may be necessary. Avoid use with 3A4 inducers.

Clinical Pearls:

Most recently approved atypical antipsychotic. Most closely similar to aripiprazole with partial D2 agonism. Manufacturer and very early data suggest D3 activity may result in negative symptom improvement.

Fun Fact:

Cariprazine was developed by a Hungarian pharmaceutical company, Gedeon Richter, which was founded in 1901 by a pharmacist. It initially processed extracts from plants to produce herbal drugs.

Bottom Line:

Cariprazine's potential claim to fame will be efficacy for negative symptoms, but the data are too preliminary to make a definitive conclusion. Beyond that, it appears to be another in a series of me-too antipsychotics, with a side effect profile heavy on EPS and akathisia as well as significant potential for weight gain.

CHLORPROMAZINE (Thorazine) Fact Sheet [G]

FDA Indications:
Psychosis; mania; nausea and vomiting; intractable hiccups.

Off-Label Uses:
Bipolar disorder; behavioral disturbances; impulse control disorders.

Dosage Forms:
- **Tablets (G):** 10 mg, 25 mg, 50 mg, 100 mg, 200 mg.
- **Injectable (G):** 25 mg/mL.

Dosage Guidance:
Schizophrenia: Start 10 mg–25 mg TID; ↑ by 20 mg–50 mg/day increments every 3–4 days to lowest effective dose. Dose range 200 mg–600 mg/day in divided doses; max FDA-approved dose 1000 mg/day.

Monitoring: ECG if cardiac disease.

Cost: $$$–$$$$ (depending on dose)

Side Effects:
- Most common: Sedation, orthostasis, tachycardia, drowsiness, dry mouth, constipation, blurred vision, prolactin elevation (sexual side effects, amenorrhea, galactorrhea).
- Serious but rare: Skin pigmentation and ocular changes (both dose related); jaundice.

Mechanism, Pharmacokinetics, and Drug Interactions:
- Dopamine D2 receptor antagonist.
- Metabolized primarily by CYP2D6, also 1A2 and 3A4. Patients who are poor metabolizers of CYP2D6 metabolize the drug more slowly, potentially increasing its effects; t ½: 23 to 37 hours.
- CYP2D6 inhibitors (eg, fluoxetine, paroxetine, quinidine) may increase chlorpromazine levels.

Clinical Pearls:
- Chlorpromazine is a low-potency conventional (typical) antipsychotic; this leads to less EPS compared to high-potency agents (eg, haloperidol, fluphenazine) and to more anticholinergic side effects compared to mid- and high-potency agents (eg, perphenazine and haloperidol, respectively).
- Extremely sedating agent and often used for this effect. Dosing limited by orthostasis and sedation.

Fun Fact:
Thorazine was developed by a French surgeon in 1948 to induce relaxation and indifference in surgical patients.

Bottom Line:
Not commonly used for core symptoms of schizophrenia; some clinicians use it at low doses (25 mg) as a non-addictive hypnotic/anxiolytic.

CLOZAPINE (Clozaril) Fact Sheet [G]

FDA Indications:

Treatment-resistant schizophrenia; reduction in risk of suicide in schizophrenia and schizoaffective disorder.

Off-Label Uses:

Treatment-resistant bipolar disorder; treatment-resistant aggression and violence.

Dosage Forms:

- **Tablets (Clozaril):** 25 mg, 100 mg (scored).
- **Tablets (G):** 25 mg, 50 mg, 100 mg, 200 mg (scored).
- **Orally disintegrating tablets (FazaClo, G):** 12.5 mg, 25 mg, 100 mg, 150 mg, 200 mg.
- **Oral suspension (Versacloz):** 50 mg/mL.

Dosage Guidance:

- Start 12.5 mg once or twice daily; ↑ gradually, in increments of 25 mg–50 mg/day to target dose 300 mg–450 mg/day by end of 2 weeks; may ↑ further in increments ≤100 mg and no more frequently than once or twice weekly. May require doses as high as 600 mg–900 mg/day; max 900 mg/day (usually in 2–3 divided doses). May take 4–6 weeks, or as long as 3–6 months, for response.
- If dosing is interrupted for ≥48 hours, must be retitrated from 12.5 mg–25 mg/day; may be increased more rapidly than initial titration, as tolerated.

Monitoring:

- Fasting glucose, lipids.
- Before starting clozapine, ensure absolute neutrophil count (ANC) >1500; for benign ethnic population (BEN) ensure two baseline ANCs ≥1000. Repeat ANC weekly for first 6 months, then every 2 weeks from 6 months to 12 months, then monthly after 12 months. If ANC falls below 1500, guidelines become complex depending on how low the value is; consult clozapine risk evaluation and mitigation strategy (REMS) (https://www.clozapinerems.com/CpmgClozapineUI/rems/pdf/resources/ANC_Table.pdf) for advice.
- Serum level monitoring can be useful; therapeutic response generally occurs between 350–450 ng/mL, though some patients may show response at lower levels. Upper limit is not well defined; increased risk of toxic effects at levels above 700 ng/mL.

Cost: $$$; oral suspension, ODT: $$$$$

Side Effects:

- Most common: Sedation, orthostatic hypotension, hypersalivation (place towel on pillow), weight gain (15–30 pound average weight gain after 1 year), constipation (risk of toxic megacolon if untreated), tachycardia (can treat with propranolol).
- Serious but rare: Potentially life-threatening agranulocytosis (1%–2%); periodic WBC testing (as above, see prescribing information for monitoring details) must occur.

Mechanism, Pharmacokinetics, and Drug Interactions:

- Dopamine D2 and serotonin 5HT2A receptor antagonist.
- Metabolized by several CYP450: 1A2, 2D6, and 3A4; t ½: 12 hours.
- Avoid use with drugs that may cause bone marrow suppression (eg, carbamazepine) and lower seizure threshold. Collapse, respiratory arrest, and cardiac arrest reported during initial clozapine treatment in patients taking benzodiazepines. Caution with P450 inhibitors and inducers.

Clinical Pearls:

- Risk of agranulocytosis greatest within first 6 months, then incidence declines but can still occur.
- Divided doses may minimize some adverse effects (eg, hypotension, seizures).
- FDA-required REMS program requires prescribers to be certified to prescribe clozapine (see www.clozapinerems.com for details).

Fun Fact:

The Quiet Room is a compelling memoir written by patient Lori Schiller, who was an early user of clozapine.

Bottom Line:

The only drug with convincing evidence based on years of clinical experience to help treatment-resistant schizophrenia. Consider using it after 2 failed trials of other antipsychotics.

FLUPHENAZINE (Prolixin) Fact Sheet [G]

FDA Indications:
Psychosis.

Off-Label Uses:
Bipolar disorder; behavioral disturbances; impulse control disorders.

Dosage Forms:
- **Tablets (G):** 1 mg, 2.5 mg, 5 mg, 10 mg.
- **Oral liquid (G):** 2.5 mg/5 mL, 5 mg/mL.
- **Injection (G):** 2.5 mg/mL.
- **Depot injection (G):** 25 mg/mL (see LAI fact sheet and table).

Dosage Guidance:
Start 1 mg–2.5 mg BID; adjust to lowest effective dose. Dose range 2.5 mg–20 mg/day divided BID; max FDA-approved dose is 40 mg/day, but doses >20 mg/day rarely more effective and difficult to tolerate.

Monitoring: No routine monitoring recommended unless clinical picture warrants.

Cost: $

Side Effects:
- Most common: EPS, headache, drowsiness, dry mouth, prolactin elevation (sexual side effects, amenorrhea, galactorrhea).
- Serious but rare: See class warnings in chapter introduction.

Mechanism, Pharmacokinetics, and Drug Interactions:
- Dopamine D2 receptor antagonist.
- Metabolized primarily by CYP2D6; t ½: 15 hours. Poor metabolizers of CYP2D6 metabolize the drug more slowly; may have increased effects.
- CYP2D6 inhibitors (eg, fluoxetine, paroxetine, quinidine) may increase fluphenazine levels.

Clinical Pearls:
- Fluphenazine is a high-potency conventional (typical) antipsychotic; this leads to more EPS compared to mid- or low-potency agents (eg, perphenazine or chlorpromazine, respectively) and to less sedation, less orthostasis, and fewer anticholinergic side effects compared to low-potency agents (eg, chlorpromazine).
- Relatively lower seizure side effect risk compared to lower-potency agents.
- Long-acting injectable decanoate formulation allows option for patients who don't take oral formation reliably.
- Availability of short-acting injectable and oral liquid formulations also allows for more flexibility in administration.

Fun Fact:
Prolixin is the most well-known brand of fluphenazine, but there was also a branded fluphenazine on the market under the name Permitil.

Bottom Line:
Fluphenazine is an effective, inexpensive typical antipsychotic with a long history of experience and use, but clinical utility is limited in some patients due to EPS.

HALOPERIDOL (Haldol) Fact Sheet [G]

FDA Indications:

Psychosis; Tourette's disorder.

Off-Label Uses:

Bipolar disorder; behavioral disturbances; impulse control disorders; delirium.

Dosage Forms:

- **Tablets (G):** 0.5 mg, 1 mg, 2 mg, 5 mg, 10 mg, 20 mg (scored).
- **Oral concentrate (G):** 2 mg/mL.
- **Injectable (G):** 5 mg/mL.
- **Depot injection (G):** 50 mg/mL and 100 mg/mL (see LAI fact sheet and table).

Dosage Guidance:

Schizophrenia: Start 1 mg–2 mg BID (5 mg BID for hospitalized patients); adjust to lowest effective dose.
Usual dose range is 5 mg–20 mg/day. Max FDA-approved dose is 100 mg/day, but doses >20 mg/day are rarely used.

Monitoring: No routine monitoring recommended unless clinical picture warrants.

Cost: $

Side Effects:

- Most common: EPS, headache, drowsiness, dry mouth, prolactin elevation (sexual side effects, amenorrhea, galactorrhea).
- Serious but rare: See class warnings in chapter introduction.

Mechanism, Pharmacokinetics, and Drug Interactions:

- Dopamine D2 receptor antagonist.
- Metabolized primarily by CYP2D6, also 3A4; t ½: 21 to 24 hours. Patients that are poor metabolizers of CYP2D6 metabolize the drug more slowly; may have increased effects.
- CYP2D6 inhibitors (eg, fluoxetine, paroxetine, quinidine) may increase haloperidol levels. May inhibit CYP2D6; caution with substrates of 2D6 as haloperidol may increase their levels and effects.

Clinical Pearls:

- Haloperidol is a high-potency conventional (typical) antipsychotic; this leads to more EPS compared to mid- or low-potency agents (eg, perphenazine or chlorpromazine, respectively) and to less sedation, less orthostasis, and fewer anticholinergic side effects compared to low-potency agents (eg, chlorpromazine).
- Relatively lower seizure side effect risk compared to lower-potency agents.
- Short-acting injectable and oral liquid formulations allow for more flexibility in administration.
- Long-acting injectable decanoate formulation allows option for patients who don't take oral formation reliably.

Fun Fact:

Haldol was discovered in 1958 by Paul Janssen, the founder of Belgian pharmaceutical company Janssen Pharmaceutica.

Bottom Line:

Haloperidol is an effective, inexpensive typical antipsychotic with a long history of experience and use, but clinical utility is limited in some patients due to EPS.

ILOPERIDONE (Fanapt) Fact Sheet

FDA Indications:
Schizophrenia.

Off-Label Uses:
Bipolar disorder; major depression; behavioral disturbances; impulse control disorders.

Dosage Forms:
Tablets: 1 mg, 2 mg, 4 mg, 6 mg, 8 mg, 10 mg, 12 mg.

Dosage Guidance:
Start 1 mg BID; ↑ to 2 mg BID on day 2 and then daily by 4 mg/day to a target dose of 6 mg–12 mg BID daily; max 12 mg BID.

Monitoring: Fasting glucose, lipids.

Cost: $$$$$

Side Effects:
- Most common: Dizziness (dose-related), dry mouth, fatigue, nasal congestion, orthostatic hypotension (can minimize by gradual dose titration), somnolence, tachycardia (dose-related), moderate weight gain.
- Serious but rare: Relatively moderate to high risk of QTc prolongation (risk is increased in patients taking potent CYP2D6 or 3A4 inhibitors, or at higher doses); avoid use in patients with bradycardia, history of MI, hypokalemia, hypomagnesemia, or concomitant use of other drugs that prolong QTc. Priapism reported rarely.

Mechanism, Pharmacokinetics, and Drug Interactions:
- Dopamine D2 and serotonin 5HT2A receptor antagonist.
- Metabolized primarily through CYP2D6 and also 3A4; t ½: 18 hours (33 hours in poor metabolizers).
- Avoid concomitant use of other drugs known to prolong the QTc interval.
- Potent inhibitors of CYP2D6 (eg, paroxetine, fluoxetine, quinidine) or 3A4 (eg, ketoconazole, clarithromycin) may increase iloperidone levels; in such cases, decrease iloperidone dose by 50%.

Clinical Pearls:
- Must follow initial titration schedule if treatment has been interrupted for >3 days.
- Minimal data regarding long-term use in schizophrenia and uses other than schizophrenia.
- Avoid use in patients with severe hepatic impairment due to potential for elevated levels leading to QT interval prolongation.

Fun Fact:
Iloperidone was initially on track for FDA approval in 2002, but its approval was delayed to 2009 due to multiple company mergers and out-licensing deals as well as the FDA's request for more data.

Bottom Line:
Not recommended as first-choice agent due to twice-daily dosing, need for titration, QT prolongation (comparable to ziprasidone), dizziness, moderate weight gain, and increases in blood sugar; and because it appears less efficacious than other antipsychotics.

LOXAPINE (Loxitane) Fact Sheet [G]

FDA Indications:
Schizophrenia; acute agitation associated with schizophrenia or acute bipolar mania.

Off-Label Uses:
Bipolar disorder; behavioral disturbances; impulse control disorders.

Dosage Forms:
- **Capsules (G):** 5 mg, 10 mg, 25 mg, 50 mg.
- **Single-use disposable inhaler (Adasuve)**, for acute agitation: 10 mg as inhalation powder.

Dosage Guidance:
- Schizophrenia: Start 10 mg BID; adjust to lowest effective dose. Dose range 60 mg–100 mg divided BID–TID; max FDA-approved dose is 250 mg/day, but doses >100 mg/day rarely used.
- Acute agitation (oral inhalation): Give 1 puff every 24 hours as needed (must be given by health care professional).

Monitoring: No routine monitoring recommended unless clinical picture warrants.

Cost: Capsule: $; inhalation: $$$

Side Effects:
- Most common: EPS, headache, drowsiness, dry mouth, prolactin elevation (sexual side effects, amenorrhea, galactorrhea), throat irritation (Adasuve).
- Serious but rare: See class warnings in chapter introduction.

Mechanism, Pharmacokinetics, and Drug Interactions:
- Dopamine D2 and serotonin 5HT2A receptor antagonist.
- Metabolized primarily by CYP2D6 and 3A4; t ½: 4–8 hours.
- Caution with inhibitors of CYP2D6 and 3A4 and inducers of 3A4; adjust dose.

Clinical Pearls:
- Loxapine is an intermediate-potency conventional (typical) antipsychotic; this leads to less EPS compared to high-potency agents (eg, haloperidol, fluphenazine) and to less sedation, less orthostasis, and fewer anticholinergic side effects compared to low-potency agents (eg, chlorpromazine).
- Loxapine belongs to the dibenzoxazepine class of antipsychotics and is structurally related to clozapine (which belongs to the chemically akin class of dibenzodiazepines). Some have argued that loxapine may behave as an atypical antipsychotic.
- The newer Adasuve oral inhalation version has the advantage of treating agitation quickly without the need for swallowing or a shot. But the risks of bronchospasm and respiratory arrest, along with the contraindication in patients with asthma, COPD, or other lung disease, make this formulation rather unappealing overall.

Fun Fact:
Loxapine is metabolized to the tetracyclic antidepressant amoxapine.

Bottom Line:
Loxapine is an effective, well-tolerated (compared to high-potency and low-potency typical antipsychotics), and inexpensive alternative to atypical antipsychotics.

LURASIDONE (Latuda) Fact Sheet

FDA Indications:
Schizophrenia (adults, adolescents 13–17); **bipolar depression** (as monotherapy and adjunct).

Off-Label Uses:
Mixed depression; treatment-resistant depression; manic episodes; impulse control disorders.

Dosage Forms:
Tablets: 20 mg, 40 mg, 60 mg, 80 mg, 120 mg.

Dosage Guidance:

- Schizophrenia (adolescents and adults): Start 40 mg QD, with food (at least 350 calories); no titration required. Usual dose 40 mg–160 mg/day. Max dose 160 mg QD (80 mg/day for adolescents).
- Bipolar depression: Start 20 mg QD, with food (at least 350 calories); no titration required. Usual dose 20 mg–120 mg/day. Max dose 120 mg QD, although doses >80 mg/day rarely more effective.

Monitoring: Fasting glucose, lipids.

Cost: $$$$$

Side Effects:

- Most common: Sedation (dose-related), akathisia (dose-related), nausea, parkinsonism, agitation.
- Serious but rare: Orthostatic hypotension and syncope reported (rarely).

Mechanism, Pharmacokinetics, and Drug Interactions:

- Dopamine D2 and serotonin 5HT2A and 5HT7 antagonist; serotonin 5HT1A partial agonist.
- Metabolized primarily through CYP450 3A4; t ½: 18 hours.
- Avoid use with medications that cause orthostasis, potent 3A4 inhibitors (eg, ketoconazole, clarithromycin), or inducers (eg, rifampin, St. John's wort, carbamazepine). Exercise caution/monitor when using in combination with moderate 3A4 inhibitors (eg, diltiazem); decrease lurasidone dose by 50% in patients taking moderate 3A4 inhibitors.

Clinical Pearls:

- Administration with food (at least 350 calories) increases bioavailability twofold and peak serum levels roughly threefold; fat content of meal is not important.
- Appears to be relatively weight-neutral and cardiometabolic parameters little affected in company-sponsored trials, although post-marketing observations have been limited.

Fun Fact:
One unique feature of Latuda is its high affinity for the 5-HT7 receptor, which has been linked to depression, learning/memory, cognition, anxiety, and pain. Unfortunately, to date, Latuda has shown no clear benefit over other atypical antipsychotics on these measures.

Bottom Line:
This drug offers some advantages, including no need for titration, once-daily dosing, relatively low-moderate metabolic profile, and relatively low QTc prolongation risk. However, its use is limited by the need to administer with ≥350 calories of food, potential for drug interactions, and side effects including sedation, akathisia, and EPS. In clinical practice, you might lump lurasidone with the other atypicals that cause little weight gain, such as aripiprazole and ziprasidone.

MOLINDONE (Moban) Fact Sheet [G]

FDA Indications:
Schizophrenia.

Off-Label Uses:
Bipolar disorder; behavioral disturbances; impulse control disorders.

Dosage Forms:
Tablets: 5 mg, 10 mg, 25 mg.

Dosage Guidance:
Start 50 mg–75 mg/day divided BID–QID; increase to 100 mg/day in 3 or 4 days. Max dose 225 mg/day divided TID–QID.

Monitoring: No routine monitoring recommended unless clinical picture warrants.

Cost: $

Side Effects:
- Most common: Sedation (dose-related), EPS, agitation.
- Serious but rare: Rare reports of leukopenia and leukocytosis.

Mechanism, Pharmacokinetics, and Drug Interactions:
- Dopamine D2 antagonist.
- Metabolized primarily through CYP450; t ½: 1.5 hours.

Clinical Pearls:
- Molindone is an intermediate-potency conventional (typical) antipsychotic; this leads to less EPS compared to high-potency agents (eg, haloperidol, fluphenazine) and to less sedation, less orthostasis, and fewer anticholinergic side effects compared to low-potency agents (eg, chlorpromazine).
- Unlike most antipsychotics, molindone has been shown to reduce weight in some patients.

Fun Fact:
In 2010, the only manufacturer of molindone in the US (as brand Moban), Endo Pharmaceuticals, announced that they would be discontinuing production because of poor sales. In December 2015, Core Pharma launched a new generic version, bringing molindone back to life.

Bottom Line:
Molindone is an effective, well-tolerated (compared to high-potency and low-potency typical antipsychotics), and inexpensive typical antipsychotic with potentially less weight gain liability than other antipsychotics.

OLANZAPINE (Zyprexa) Fact Sheet [G]

FDA Indications:

Schizophrenia (adults and children ≥13 years); acute or mixed **bipolar** I manic episodes, as monotherapy or adjunct (adults and children ≥13 years); maintenance treatment of bipolar disorder; **bipolar depression** (with fluoxetine, sold as Symbyax, adults and children ≥10 years); **treatment-resistant unipolar depression** (with fluoxetine); **acute agitation** in schizophrenia and bipolar mania (injectable form).

Off-Label Uses:

Behavioral disturbances; impulse control disorders.

Dosage Forms:

- **Tablets (G):** 2.5 mg, 5 mg, 7.5 mg, 10 mg, 15 mg, 20 mg.
- **Orally disintegrating tablets (G):** 5 mg, 10 mg, 15 mg, 20 mg.
- **IM injection (G):** 10 mg.
- **Depot injection:** 210 mg, 300 mg, 405 mg (see LAI fact sheet and table).
- **Fixed combination capsules with fluoxetine (G):** 3/25 mg, 6/25 mg, 12/25 mg, 6/50 mg, 12/50 mg olanzapine/fluoxetine.

Dosage Guidance:

- Schizophrenia, bipolar disorder, depression (adults): Start most patients at 5 mg–10 mg QD; may ↑ by 5 mg QD, in weekly increments, to target dose 10 mg–20 mg QD.
- Acute mania (adults): Start 10 mg–15 mg QD; may ↑ by 5 mg daily, in 24-hour increments, to target dose 10 mg–20 mg QD.
- Max approved dose: 20 mg/day, although doses up to 30 mg–50 mg/day have been used.
- Bipolar depression (Symbyax, fixed combination with fluoxetine) (adults): Start 6/25 mg QPM, ↑ as indicated to target dose 6 mg–12 mg/25 mg–50 mg olanzapine/fluoxetine.

Monitoring: Fasting glucose, lipids.

Cost: $; ODT: $$; combination with fluoxetine: $$$

Side Effects:

- Most common: Somnolence (dose-related), dry mouth (dose-related), constipation, weight gain (up to 40% incidence; may be substantial; 10 to 30 pounds weight gain is common), increased appetite, EPS (dose-related).
- Serious but rare: Rare but potentially fatal drug reaction with eosinophilia and systemic symptoms (DRESS) possible; often starts as rash that may spread, fever, swollen lymph nodes, and elevated eosinophils.

Mechanism, Pharmacokinetics, and Drug Interactions:

- Dopamine D2 and serotonin 5HT2A receptor antagonist.
- Metabolized by CYP450 1A2, 2D6 (minor), and direct glucuronidation; t ½: 1 to 2 days.
- CYP1A2 inducers (eg, carbamazepine, ritonavir, smoking) may reduce olanzapine levels by 50%; CYP1A2 inhibitors (eg, fluvoxamine) may increase olanzapine bioavailability by 50%–100%. Adjust olanzapine dosing in presence of 1A2 inducers or inhibitors.

Clinical Pearl:

Use in children and adolescents may result in increased weight gain and sedation, as well as greater increases in LDL cholesterol, total cholesterol, triglycerides, prolactin, and liver transaminase levels when compared to adults.

Fun Fact:

Olanzapine has been studied and is used for chemotherapy-induced nausea and vomiting.

Bottom Line:

Good efficacy, particularly in acute schizophrenia and bipolar mania, once-daily dosing, and low risk of QTc interval prolongation make this an appealing drug. However, its high risk for weight gain and metabolic complications make it a second-line choice for many.

PALIPERIDONE (Invega) Fact Sheet [G]

FDA Indications:

Schizophrenia in adults and children ≥12 years; **schizoaffective disorder**.

Off-Label Uses:

Bipolar disorder; behavioral disturbances; impulse control disorders.

Dosage Forms:

- **Controlled release tablets (G):** 1.5 mg, 3 mg, 6 mg, 9 mg (not breakable).
- **Monthly depot injection (Invega Sustenna):** 39 mg, 78 mg, 117 mg, 156 mg, 234 mg (see LAI fact sheet and table).
- **Every-3-month depot injection (Invega Trinza):** 273 mg, 410 mg, 546 mg, 819 mg (see LAI fact sheet and table).

Dosage Guidance:

- Schizophrenia/schizoaffective disorder (adults): Start 6 mg QAM, which may be the effective dose; if required, may ↑ by 3 mg/day at intervals of >5 days to max 12 mg/day.
- Schizophrenia (adolescents): Start 3 mg QAM, ↑ by 3 mg/day at intervals of >5 days to max 6 mg/day (<51 kg) or 12 mg/day (≥51 kg).
- Paliperidone 3 mg, 6 mg, 9 mg, and 12 mg roughly equivalent to 1–2 mg, 2–4 mg, 4–6 mg, and 6–8 mg risperidone, respectively.

Monitoring: Fasting glucose, lipids; prolactin if symptoms.

Cost: $$$$

Side Effects:

- Most common: Akathisia, EPS (dose-related), tremor, tachycardia, insomnia, somnolence (especially adolescents), weight gain, orthostatic hypotension, headache, prolactin elevation.
- Serious but rare: Modest increase in QTc interval. Orthostatic hypotension and syncope reported. Rarely, controlled release tablet may get caught in GI tract and cause obstructive symptoms in patients with known strictures; avoid use in patients with severe, preexisting GI narrowing (either pathologic or iatrogenic). Esophageal dysmotility and aspiration possible; use caution in patients at risk for aspiration pneumonia (eg, those with advanced Alzheimer's dementia).

Mechanism, Pharmacokinetics, and Drug Interactions:

- Dopamine D2 and serotonin 5HT2A receptor antagonist.
- Not metabolized by liver; t ½: 23 hours.
- Avoid use with drugs known to prolong the QT interval or to cause orthostasis. Paliperidone is the principal active metabolite of risperidone; therefore, avoid use with risperidone. Minimal drug interactions.

Clinical Pearls:

- Warn your patients that they may find what looks like intact capsules in their stool. These are actually empty "ghost pills." They are caused by the fact that Invega (and Concerta, see fact sheet) is an extended release tablet based on the OROS osmotic delivery system: Water from the GI tract enters through a semipermeable membrane coating the tablet, causing the drug to be expelled through laser-drilled holes in the coating. The shell is nonabsorbable and will be expelled in the stool.
- Swallow whole, with fluids; do not chew, divide, or crush.
- Studies suggest paliperidone is not highly effective in acute mania, either as monotherapy or in combination with lithium or valproate.
- Along with risperidone, causes the most EPS and hyperprolactinemia of all the atypicals.

Fun Fact:

First drug with FDA approval for schizoaffective disorder, allowing Janssen to carve out a new marketing niche and separate this drug from its competitors (at least from a commercial and marketing perspective).

Bottom Line:

Invega looks like risperidone without drug-drug interactions, but with more QT interval prolongation, more tachycardia, possibly more EPS, and the same amount of hyperprolactinemia. These significant disadvantages make it a second-line option. The option to transition to a long-acting injectable without oral overlap does make Invega appealing for some patients.

PERPHENAZINE (Trilafon) Fact Sheet [G]

FDA Indications:
Schizophrenia; severe nausea and vomiting.

Off-Label Uses:
Bipolar disorder; behavioral disturbances; impulse control disorders.

Dosage Forms:
Tablets (G): 2 mg, 4 mg, 8 mg, 16 mg.

Dosage Guidance:
Schizophrenia: Start 4 mg–8 mg TID (8 mg–16 mg BID–QID for hospitalized patients); adjust to lowest effective dose. Dose range 8 mg–16 mg BID–QID; max FDA-approved dose for non-hospitalized patients is 24 mg/day, but hospitalized psychotic patients may be dosed up to 64 mg/day.

Monitoring: No routine monitoring recommended unless clinical picture warrants.

Cost: $$

Side Effects:
- Most common: EPS, headache, drowsiness, dry mouth, prolactin elevation (sexual side effects, amenorrhea, galactorrhea).
- Serious but rare: Tachycardia (especially with sudden marked increase in dose).

Mechanism, Pharmacokinetics, and Drug Interactions:
- Dopamine D2 receptor antagonist.
- Metabolized primarily by CYP2D6; t ½: 9 to 12 hours. May inhibit CYP2D6. Poor metabolizers of CYP2D6 metabolize the drug more slowly; may have increased effects.
- CYP2D6 inhibitors (eg, fluoxetine, paroxetine, quinidine) may increase perphenazine levels. Caution with substrates of 2D6 as perphenazine may increase their levels and effects.

Clinical Pearls:
- Perphenazine is an intermediate-potency conventional (typical) antipsychotic; this leads to less EPS compared to high-potency agents (eg, haloperidol, fluphenazine) and to less sedation, less orthostasis, and fewer anticholinergic side effects compared to low-potency agents (eg, chlorpromazine).
- Fewer metabolic effects (weight gain, glucose, lipids) than some antipsychotics.
- Based on 18-month, randomized trial of 1,493 patients with schizophrenia (CATIE trial), perphenazine appears similar in efficacy and EPS compared to atypical antipsychotics (olanzapine, quetiapine, risperidone, ziprasidone).

Fun Fact:
Perphenazine has long been available in a formulation with amitriptyline (a tricyclic antidepressant) called Triavil. This combination antipsychotic/antidepressant was first available in 1965, foreshadowing the next such combination drug (Symbyax) by 38 years.

Bottom Line:
Effective, well-tolerated, and inexpensive alternative to atypical antipsychotics.

PIMAVANSERIN (Nuplazid) Fact Sheet

FDA Indications:
Hallucinations and delusions associated with Parkinson's disease psychosis.

Off-Label Uses:
Too new to tell.

Dosage Forms:
Tablets: 17 mg.

Dosage Guidance:
Start and continue with 34 mg (2 tablets) once daily (no titration).

Monitoring: Fasting glucose, lipids.

Cost: $$$$$

Side Effects:
- Most common: Nausea, peripheral edema, confusion.
- Serious but rare: QT prolongation (dose-related; mean prolongation of 5–8 msec at usual dose); class warning regarding increased mortality in elderly.

Mechanism, Pharmacokinetics, and Drug Interactions:
- Atypical antipsychotic with combination of inverse agonist and antagonist activity at 5-HT2A and, less so, at 5-HT2C receptors.
- Metabolized by CYP3A4 and 3A5; t ½: 57 hours (200 hours for active metabolite).
- Caution with potent inhibitors or inducers of 3A4 (adjust dose by 50%). Avoid use with other medications that may increase QT interval.

Clinical Pearls:
- FDA approval based on one 6-week placebo-controlled outpatient study of 185 patients that showed only modest (but statistically significant) improvement in hallucinations and delusions compared to placebo.
- The study didn't find any difference (improvement or worsening) in motor function between those who received Nuplazid or placebo.
- Two previous studies did not show efficacy.

Fun Fact:
Unlike other atypical antipsychotics, Nuplazid does not have effects on dopamine receptors, and this may contribute to the finding that it doesn't worsen motor symptoms in Parkinson's.

Bottom Line:
Hallucinations and delusions occur in the later stages of Parkinson's and are sometimes worsened by the dopaminergic medications used to treat the disorder. Quetiapine (Seroquel) has generally been considered to be the antipsychotic least likely to worsen Parkinson's disease motor symptoms. Nuplazid is now the only approved medication for this indication, but we do not yet know if it has any efficacy advantages over quetiapine. The fact that it does not cause weight gain, however, is a side effect advantage.

QUETIAPINE (Seroquel) Fact Sheet [G]

FDA Indications:

Schizophrenia (adults and children ≥13 years); **bipolar,** manic/mixed (adults and children ≥10 years); **bipolar depression;** maintenance treatment for bipolar; **major depression,** as adjunct.

Off-Label Uses:

Insomnia; anxiety disorders; behavioral disturbances; impulse control disorders.

Dosage Forms:

- **Tablets (G):** 25 mg, 50 mg, 100 mg, 200 mg, 300 mg, 400 mg.
- **ER tablets (G):** 50 mg, 150 mg, 200 mg, 300 mg, 400 mg.

Dosage Guidance:

- Schizophrenia (adults): Start 25 mg BID or 300 mg XR QHS. Target dose: 400–800 mg/day.
- Bipolar (adults): Start 50 mg BID or 300 mg XR QHS. Target dose: 400–800 mg/day (mania, maintenance), 300 mg/day (depression).
- Adolescents: Start 25 mg BID or 50 mg XR QHS, increase to 100 mg/day (IR divided BID, XR taken QHS) on day 2, then increase by 100 mg/day daily to target dose 400–600 mg/day (mania) or 400–600 mg/day (schizophrenia).
- Depression: Start 50 mg IR/XR QHS. Target dose: 150–300 mg/day.
- For all indications: May ↑ dose by 50 mg–100 mg/day increments, given in divided doses, every 1–4 days (or as much as 300 mg/day XR increments in intervals of >1 day) to target dose.
- Max daily dose in adults: 800 mg/day.
- Consider dosing slower and lower in pediatric, elderly, or debilitated patients.

Monitoring: Fasting glucose, lipids.

Cost: IR: $; ER: $$$$

Side Effects:

- Most common: Somnolence, hypotension, dry mouth, dizziness, constipation, weight gain, fatigue.
- Serious but rare: Orthostatic hypotension, particularly at high dose or with rapid titration.

Mechanism, Pharmacokinetics, and Drug Interactions:

- Dopamine D2 and serotonin 5HT2A receptor antagonist.
- Metabolized by CYP3A4; t ½: 6 hours (XR: 7 hours).
- Avoid or use caution with agents that may cause additional orthostasis. CYP3A4 inducers (eg, carbamazepine) may lower quetiapine levels; CYP3A4 inhibitors (eg, erythromycin, ketoconazole) may increase quetiapine levels. Adjust quetiapine dose in presence of CYP3A4 inducers or inhibitors.

Clinical Pearls:

- Swallow XR tablet whole; do not break, crush, or chew; switch between IR and XR at the same total daily dose; dose adjustments may be necessary based on response and tolerability.
- If patient discontinues drug >1 week, retitrate dose as with initial therapy.
- Quetiapine abuse has been reported, particularly in incarcerated populations.

Fun Fact:

Cataracts developed in initial studies with beagle dogs; human studies have not shown an association. However, the label still recommends a slit-lamp exam every 6 months.

Bottom Line:

Low risk for EPS and a broad spectrum of efficacy make this an appealing first-choice agent. However, sedation, weight gain, and orthostasis may limit use. Dosing at bedtime, or switching to XR, may help reduce daytime sedation.

RISPERIDONE (Risperdal) Fact Sheet [G]

FDA Indications:

Schizophrenia (adults and children ≥13 years); **bipolar disorder**, **manic/mixed** (adults and children ≥10 years); **irritability symptoms of autism** (children ≥5 years).

Off-Label Uses:

Bipolar depression; behavioral disturbances; impulse control disorders; Tourette syndrome.

Dosage Forms:

- **Tablets (G):** 0.25 mg, 0.5 mg, 1 mg, 2 mg, 3 mg, 4 mg.
- **Oral solution (G):** 1 mg/mL.
- **Orally disintegrating tablets (Risperdal M-Tab, G):** 0.25 mg, 0.5 mg, 1 mg, 2 mg, 3 mg, 4 mg.
- **Depot injection (Risperdal Consta):** 12.5 mg, 25 mg, 37.5 mg, 50 mg (see LAI fact sheet and table).

Dosage Guidance:

- Schizophrenia, bipolar (adults): Start 1 mg BID; may ↑ by 1 mg–2 mg/day at intervals ≥24 hours to a recommended dosage range 4 mg–6 mg/day; may be given as a single daily dose once maintenance dose achieved. Max approved dose is 16 mg/day, but daily dosages >6 mg provide no additional benefit, only higher risk for EPS, which is dose-dependent.
- Children, elderly, first-episode psychosis: Lower initial dosages (eg, 0.5 mg–1 mg daily) and slower titration to initial target dose of 2 mg daily.
- Autism (children ≥5 years): If <15 kg (33 lbs), use with caution. For 15 kg–20 kg (33 lbs–44 lbs), start 0.25 mg/day, ↑ to 0.5 mg/day after ≥4 days. If response insufficient, may ↑ by 0.25 mg/day in ≥2-week intervals; give QD or BID. For ≥20 kg (44 lbs), start 0.5 mg/day; may ↑ to 1 mg/day after ≥4 days. If response insufficient, may ↑ dose by 0.5 mg/day in ≥2-week intervals; give QD or BID.
- Bipolar mania or schizophrenia (children): Start 0.5 mg QD; ↑ in increments of 0.5 mg–1 mg/day at intervals ≥24 hours to target dose of 2 mg–3 mg/day; doses >3 mg/day do not confer additional benefit and are associated with increased side effects.

Monitoring: Fasting glucose, lipids; prolactin if symptoms.

Cost: $; ODT: $$–$$$ (depending on dose)

Side Effects:

- Most common: EPS, somnolence (particularly in children), anxiety, constipation, nausea, dyspepsia, dizziness, rhinitis, prolactin elevation, weight gain.
- Serious but rare: Orthostatic hypotension may occur, particularly at higher doses or with rapid titration. Hyperprolactinemia with clinical symptoms (sexual side effects, galactorrhea, amenorrhea).

Mechanism, Pharmacokinetics, and Drug Interactions:

- Dopamine D2 and serotonin 5HT2A receptor antagonist.
- Metabolized by CYP2D6; t ½: 20 hours.
- CYP2D6 inhibitors (eg, fluoxetine, paroxetine, quinidine) may increase effects of risperidone; reduce risperidone dose. Carbamazepine reduces levels and effects of risperidone; may need to double risperidone dose.

Clinical Pearls:

- Along with paliperidone, causes the most EPS and hyperprolactinemia of all the atypicals.
- When reinitiating after discontinuation, initial titration schedule should be followed.

Fun Fact:

Risperdal M-tabs are marketed in other countries as Risperdal Quicklets.

Bottom Line:

Risperidone has been widely used and is often used first-line. At higher doses (>4 mg/day), risperidone may not provide some of the putative advantages of other atypical antipsychotics, particularly with regard to side effects.

THIORIDAZINE (Mellaril) Fact Sheet [G]

FDA Indications:
Schizophrenia (not for first-line use).

Off-Label Uses:
Anxiety, insomnia.

Dosage Forms:
Tablets (G): 10 mg, 25 mg, 50 mg, 100 mg.

Dosage Guidance:
Start 50 mg–100 mg TID; adjust to lowest effective dose. Dose range 200 mg–800 mg/day divided BID–QID; max FDA-approved dose is 800 mg/day due to ocular pigmentation at high doses.

Monitoring: ECG if cardiac disease.

Cost: $

Side Effects:
- Most common: EPS, headache, sedation, drowsiness, dry mouth, constipation, blurred vision, dizziness, prolactin elevation (sexual side effects, amenorrhea, galactorrhea).
- Serious but rare: QT prolongation and torsades de pointes (highest risk of all antipsychotics); ocular pigmentation and degenerative retinopathies.

Mechanism, Pharmacokinetics, and Drug Interactions:
- Dopamine D2 receptor antagonist.
- Metabolized primarily by CYP2D6; t ½: 24 hours. May inhibit CYP2D6. Poor metabolizers of CYP2D6 metabolize the drug more slowly; may have increased effects.
- CYP2D6 inhibitors (eg, fluoxetine, paroxetine, quinidine) may increase thioridazine levels. Caution with substrates of 2D6 as thioridazine may increase their levels and effects.

Clinical Pearls:
- Thioridazine is a low-potency conventional (typical) antipsychotic; this leads to less EPS and to more sedation, orthostasis, and anticholinergic side effects compared to high-potency agents (eg, haloperidol, fluphenazine).
- Efficacy has not been studied in refractory schizophrenia, but thioridazine is indicated only for and should be reserved for use only in patients who have failed to respond to other medications. This is due to the significant risks associated with thioridazine, particularly QT prolongation.

Fun Fact:
Thioridazine can kill antibiotic-resistant bacteria such as *Staphylococcus aureus* (including MRSA) and extensively drug-resistant (XDR) *Mycobacterium tuberculosis*. Researchers are studying how thioridazine does this (latest studies show a weakening of bacterial cell walls) in order to develop drugs that can target resistant bacteria.

Bottom Line:
Too risky to use for the majority of patients.

THIOTHIXENE (Navane) Fact Sheet [G]

FDA Indications:
Schizophrenia.

Off-Label Uses:
Bipolar disorder; behavioral disturbances; impulse control disorders.

Dosage Forms:
Capsules (G): 1 mg, 2 mg, 5 mg, 10 mg, 20 mg.

Dosage Guidance:
Start 2 mg TID–5 mg BID; adjust to lowest effective dose. Usual dose range 20 mg–30 mg/day divided BID–TID; max FDA-approved dose is 60 mg/day, but doses >40 mg/day are rarely used.

Monitoring: No routine monitoring recommended unless clinical picture warrants.

Cost: $$

Side Effects:
- Most common: EPS, headache, drowsiness, dry mouth, prolactin elevation (sexual side effects, amenorrhea, galactorrhea).
- Serious but rare: See class warnings in chapter introduction.

Mechanism, Pharmacokinetics, and Drug Interactions:
- Dopamine D2 receptor antagonist.
- Metabolized primarily by CYP1A2; t ½: 34 hours.
- Smoking status may affect thiothixene metabolism as smoking is a potent 1A2 inducer; smokers may need higher doses.

Clinical Pearl:
Thiothixene is a high-potency conventional (typical) antipsychotic; this leads to more EPS compared to mid- and low-potency agents (eg, perphenazine or chlorpromazine, respectively) and to less sedation, less orthostasis, and fewer anticholinergic side effects compared to low-potency agents (eg, chlorpromazine).

Fun Fact:
Pfizer developed thiothixene in the 1960s, and the drug was found to be an effective antidepressant, as well as an antipsychotic. For commercial reasons, the company chose to market it for schizophrenia rather than depression.

Bottom Line:
When using a high-potency typical antipsychotic, most will choose haloperidol or fluphenazine because of greater familiarity with those agents and a range of formulation options (eg, liquid, injectable, long-acting).

TRIFLUOPERAZINE (Stelazine) Fact Sheet [G]

FDA Indications:
Schizophrenia; non-psychotic anxiety.

Off-Label Uses:
Bipolar disorder; behavioral disturbances; impulse control disorders.

Dosage Forms:
Tablets (G): 1 mg, 2 mg, 5 mg, 10 mg.

Dosage Guidance:
Schizophrenia: Start 1 mg–2 mg BID; adjust to lowest effective dose. Usual dose range 5 mg–10 mg BID; max FDA-approved dose 40 mg/day.

Monitoring: No routine monitoring recommended unless clinical picture warrants.

Cost: $$

Side Effects:
- Most common: EPS, headache, drowsiness, dry mouth, prolactin elevation (sexual side effects, amenorrhea, galactorrhea).
- Serious but rare: See class warnings in chapter introduction.

Mechanism, Pharmacokinetics, and Drug Interactions:
- Dopamine D2 receptor antagonist.
- Metabolized primarily by CYP1A2; t ½: 18 hours.
- Smoking status may affect trifluoperazine metabolism as smoking is a potent 1A2 inducer; smokers may need higher doses.

Clinical Pearls:
- Trifluoperazine is a high-potency conventional (typical) antipsychotic; this leads to more EPS compared to mid- and low-potency agents (eg, perphenazine or chlorpromazine, respectively) and to less sedation, less orthostasis, and fewer anticholinergic side effects compared to low-potency agents (eg, chlorpromazine).
- Trifluoperazine was FDA-approved for non-psychotic anxiety at doses of no more than 6 mg/day used for no more than 12 weeks, but it is no longer used for this indication.

Fun Fact:
Stelazine was marketed with the tagline slogan "Calm, but still alert."

Bottom Line:
When using a high-potency typical antipsychotic, most will choose haloperidol or fluphenazine because of greater familiarity with those agents and a range of formulation options (eg, liquid, injectable, long-acting).

ZIPRASIDONE (Geodon) Fact Sheet [G]

FDA Indications:

Schizophrenia; bipolar disorder, acute treatment of manic/mixed episode; maintenance treatment of **bipolar disorder** as adjunct; **acute agitation** in patients with schizophrenia (IM only).

Off-Label Uses:

Bipolar disorder; behavioral disturbances; impulse control disorders.

Dosage Forms:

- **Capsules (G):** 20 mg, 40 mg, 60 mg, 80 mg.
- **Injection (Geodon):** 20 mg/mL.

Dosage Guidance:

- Schizophrenia, bipolar disorder: Start 20 mg BID (40 mg BID for acute mania) with meals for 2 to 3 days; ↑ by 40 mg/day increments; can usually ↑ rather quickly to target dose 60 mg–80 mg BID. Max approved dose is 160 mg/day, though can go higher in some patients; there are some safety data for doses up to 320 mg/day.
- Schizophrenia, acute agitation (IM injection): 10 mg Q2 hours or 20 mg Q4 hours; max 40 mg/day. Replace with oral therapy as soon as possible.

Monitoring: Fasting glucose, lipids; ECG if cardiac disease.

Cost: $

Side Effects:

- Most common: Somnolence, dizziness, akathisia, rash (5%).
- Serious but rare: May result in minor QTc prolongation (dose-related; 10 msec at 160 mg/day). Clinically relevant prolongation (>500 msec) rare (0.06%) and less than placebo (0.23%). Significant QTc prolongation has been associated with the development of malignant ventricular arrhythmias (torsades de pointes) and sudden death. Avoid in patients with hypokalemia, hypomagnesemia, bradycardia, persistent QTc intervals >500 msec, or those receiving other drugs that prolong QTc interval. Patients with symptoms of dizziness, palpitations, or syncope should receive further cardiac evaluation. Drug reaction with eosinophilia and systemic symptoms (DRESS) has been reported with ziprasidone exposure. DRESS begins as a rash that can spread all over the body; it may also include swollen lymph nodes, fever, and damage to organs such as the heart, liver, pancreas, or kidneys, and is sometimes fatal; discontinue ziprasidone if DRESS is suspected.

Mechanism, Pharmacokinetics, and Drug Interactions:

- Dopamine D2 and serotonin 5HT2A receptor antagonist.
- Metabolized in liver principally by aldehyde oxidase; less than one-third of clearance mediated by CYP450: CYP3A4 (major), and CYP1A2 (minor); t ½: 7 hours.
- Avoid use with other drugs that prolong QTc interval.

Clinical Pearls:

- Administer twice daily, ideally with meals; ingestion of several hundred calories is necessary to increase absorption up to twofold.
- Causes less weight gain than clozapine, olanzapine, quetiapine, or risperidone.
- Average increase in QTc is greater than any other atypicals, although not much more than for quetiapine. Post-marketing surveillance has shown one or two instances of torsades de pointes possibly related to ziprasidone use.

Fun Fact:

The brand name Geodon has been suggested to bring to mind the phrase "down (don) to earth (geo)," referring to the goals of the medication.

Bottom Line:

Ziprasidone has an appealing weight and metabolic profile, but dosage titration, twice-daily dosing, and wide range for target dose make this agent more cumbersome to use. The QTc interval prolongation risk is not clinically important for the majority of patients, but use caution if risk factors exist (bradycardia, low potassium or magnesium).

LONG-ACTING INJECTABLE (LAI) Antipsychotics

INTRODUCTION: DO LAIs WORK?

These formulations used to be known as "depot" antipsychotics, but the powers that be have renamed them "long-acting injectables" (LAIs), presumably to help remove some of the stigma associated with their use.

Theoretically, LAIs are great solutions for patients who are at high risk of relapse when they stop taking their medications. Indeed, these are the patients in whom we usually entertain the possibility of prescribing an injectable. For example, I have a patient who does quite well when he takes his Clozaril, but when he stops, he ends up isolating himself in his subsidized apartment, the shades drawn, frozen in a series of paranoid delusions. Eventually, someone calls the police and he is involuntarily committed to the hospital, where he is put back on meds and does well—until the cycle repeats itself. Why isn't he on LAIs? Because he refuses to take them. He hates injections. He doesn't want to feel controlled by a medication that stays in his system. This is an example of why it's hard to demonstrate in controlled trials that LAIs prevent relapse any better than orals.

The most recent and largest meta-analysis analyzed 21 randomized controlled trials in which patients with schizophrenia were randomly assigned to either LAIs or orals. There was no difference between the formulations in relapse rates. The exception was that older studies done prior to 1992 showed a benefit of first-generation LAIs (mainly Prolixin Decanoate) over first-generation orals (Kishimoto T et al, *Schiz Bull* 2014;40(1):192–213).

But as usual with research, there are complications in interpreting these studies. While randomized controlled trials are typically the gold standard, in this case, they may not be generalizable to the kinds of patients for whom we would recommend LAIs. Such trials invite all patients, whether or not they are at high risk of non-adherence to pills. In the real world, we would rarely offer LAIs to our patients who are taking their oral medication as directed, but rather to patients who have a history of frequent relapse due to non-adherence.

In fact, naturalistic studies (also known as observational studies) tend to be much more positive about LAIs. These studies make no effort to recruit or to randomize patients to different treatment arms. Instead, they identify patients with schizophrenia in real-world settings who were switched from orals to LAIs by their doctors. The reasons for the switches are typically what you'd expect—poor adherence and poor results on orals. A meta-analysis of 25 of these studies, involving 5,940 patients, found that switching these patients to LAIs strongly decreased the number of hospitalizations (Kishimoto T et al, *J Clin Psychiatry* 2013;74(10):957–965).

The bottom line is that common sense wins the day. Patients who do poorly on pills because of non-adherence are likely to do better on LAIs—if you can get them to agree to get the needle.

With this long-winded introduction out of the way, we can finally get to what you've been waiting for—a comparison of the specific advantages and disadvantages of the many LAIs currently marketed.

DECIDING AMONG THE LAIs

General Notes on LAIs

- It's best to choose an LAI version of an oral medication that your patient has already taken, so that you can be more confident that the agent is effective and tolerable.
- Be patient. The full therapeutic effect of LAIs can take longer than orals—ie, several months. Don't adjust the LAI dose prematurely.
- Consider oral overlap. Agents differ on how quickly you can titrate up the dose. This is important because for those requiring gradual titration, patients will need oral pills to make sure they have a decent serum level right away. This process is called the "oral overlap" and it has two disadvantages. First, it makes the process of dosing a bit more complex (not a huge deal); second, if the patient is refusing to take oral meds (but accepting an injection, either under court order or voluntarily), you'll have to choose a different LAI or risk a decompensation while waiting for levels to become therapeutic.
- *Never* initiate an LAI on a patient who has a history of neuroleptic malignant syndrome (NMS) on any antipsychotic. That's just asking for trouble.

LAI Options

- There's a pretty comprehensive table on the following pages that reports, for each LAI, the **FDA indication(s), medication names, costs, available strengths, dosing information,** and **pharmacokinetics** (need for oral overlap and dosing interval). But first, we'll give you a shorthand version of the most relevant **clinical pearls** below:

Typical antipsychotics

- **Fluphenazine (Prolixin Decanoate)**—Dosed every 2 weeks. Injections are painful. Cheap, but relatively high risk of EPS and TD. Oral overlap required.
- **Haloperidol (Haldol Decanoate)**—Dosed monthly. As cheap as Prolixin, and since it's dosed less often and the pharmacokinetics are more predictable, it's generally the better choice among FGAs. Oral overlap required, although some use a "loading dose" method (20 times oral dose, followed by 10–15 times oral dose in subsequent months) which requires no oral overlap (Ereshefsky L et al, *Hosp Community Psychiatry* 1993;44(12):1155–1161).

Atypical antipsychotics

- **Aripiprazole (Abilify Maintena)**—Dosed monthly. Oral overlap required for 14 days. Deltoid or gluteal injection. Expensive. Good side effect profile.
- **Aripiprazole lauroxil (Aristada)**—Dosed monthly, every 6 weeks, or every 2 months. Smallest dose (441 mg monthly) may be given deltoid or gluteal; other doses must be given gluteal. Dosing interval flexibility makes this formulation appealing, although oral overlap is required for 21 days. Expensive. Good side effect profile.
- **Olanzapine (Zyprexa Relprevv)**—Dosed either every 2 weeks or monthly, depending on the dose needed. May be the worst choice among all LAIs for multiple reasons. High potential for weight gain. There's a small risk of a post-injection delirium/sedation syndrome, occurring in less than 1% of patients, caused by accidental intravascular injection. For this reason, you have to give the injection at a registered health care facility where patients can be continuously monitored for at least 3 hours after the injection. Restricted use requires physician and facility registration, and additional paperwork with Eli Lilly's program. High cost, restriction of use, monitoring requirement, and risk of adverse outcome all limit use severely. Gluteal injection only. Expensive. No oral overlap.
- **Paliperidone palmitate monthly (Invega Sustenna)**—Monthly dosing. Less painful injection than Risperdal Consta or Zyprexa Relprevv. No oral overlap required; need for 2 separate loading injections makes initiation a bit more complicated. First 2 doses deltoid; subsequent doses may be deltoid or gluteal. Expensive. No oral overlap and potential to transition to every-3-month formulation are appealing features.
- **Paliperidone palmitate every 3 months (Invega Trinza)**—Every-3-month dosing, but your patient must have done well on monthly injections of Sustenna for at least 4 months before switching to Trinza. Deltoid or gluteal injection. Must shake syringe vigorously for at least 15 seconds to ensure uniform suspension of long-acting particles and prevent clogging in needle. Expensive. No oral overlap.
- **Risperidone (Risperdal Consta)**—Every-2-week dosing. A 3-week oral overlap and the need for a refrigerated solution make this LAI more cumbersome to use than some of its competitors. Painful injection. Must shake for at least 10 seconds to ensure uniform suspension of microspheres. Deltoid or gluteal. Expensive.

TABLE 7: Long-Acting Injectable Antipsychotics

Generic Name (Brand Name) Year FDA Approved *[G] denotes generic availability*	Relevant FDA Indication(s)	Available Strengths	Oral Overlap	Dosing Interval	Initial Dosing	Maintenance Dose	Cost for Monthly Supply at Average Dose (July 2017)
Typical Antipsychotics							
Fluphenazine decanoate [G] (Prolixin Decanoate[1]) 1972	Schizophrenia	25 mg/mL	Continue total oral dose for 2–3 days, then ↓ by 50% increments every 2–3 days until discontinued (by next injection)	2 weeks	1.25 X total daily oral dose Q2–3 weeks	Increase in increments of 12.5 mg; do not exceed 100 mg per dose	$ [G]
Haloperidol decanoate [G] (Haldol Decanoate) 1986	Schizophrenia	50 mg/mL and 100 mg/mL	For 7 days, give usual oral dose, then ↓ by 50% weekly for 2 weeks, then discontinue	4 weeks	10–15 X total oral daily dose Q4 weeks. First dose should be ≤100 mg; if higher dose needed, give remainder in 1–2 weeks.	Continue 10–15 X total oral daily dose Q4 weeks	$ [G] $$$$ Haldol Dec
Atypical Antipsychotics							
Aripiprazole (Abilify Maintena) 2013	Schizophrenia Bipolar disorder	300 mg and 400 mg vials	For 14 days	4 weeks	400 mg Q4 weeks	400 mg Q4 weeks; decrease to 300 mg Q4 weeks if side effects	$$$$$
Aripiprazole lauroxil (Aristada) 2015	Schizophrenia	441 mg, 662 mg, 882 mg, 1064 mg	For 21 days	Monthly, every 6 weeks, or every 2 months	441 mg, 662 mg, or 882 mg monthly (equiv to 10, 15, and 20 mg/day); or 882 mg every 6 weeks (15 mg/day); or 1064 mg every 2 months (15 mg/day).	Continue initial dosing or adjust based on clinical response	$$$$$
Olanzapine (Zyprexa Relprevv) 2009	Schizophrenia	210, 300, and 405 mg vials	No overlap	2–4 weeks	10 mg/day oral: 210 mg Q2 weeks x 4 doses or 405 mg Q4 weeks x 2 doses; 15 mg/day oral: 300 mg Q2 weeks x 4 doses; 20 mg/day oral: 300 mg Q2 weeks	10 mg/day oral: 150 mg Q2 weeks or 300 mg Q4 weeks; 15 mg/day oral: 210 mg Q2 weeks or 405 mg Q4 weeks; 20 mg/day oral: 300 mg Q2 weeks; Maximum dose: 300 mg Q2 weeks or 405 mg Q4 weeks	$$$$$
Paliperidone palmitate (Invega Sustenna) 2009	Schizophrenia Schizoaffective disorder (monotherapy or adjunct)	39, 78, 117, 156, and 234 mg in prefilled syringes	No overlap	4 weeks	234 mg IM in deltoid, then 156 mg 1 week later	117 mg 3 weeks after 2nd dose then Q month; may adjust monthly dose (maintenance given deltoid or gluteal) Approx. equivalence: 3 mg oral: 39 mg–78 mg 6 mg oral: 117 mg 12 mg oral: 234 mg	$$$$$

[1]brand discontinued; available as generic only

Generic Name (Brand Name) Year FDA Approved *[G] denotes generic availability*	Relevant FDA Indication(s)	Available Strengths	Oral Overlap	Dosing Interval	Initial Dosing	Maintenance Dose	Cost for Monthly Supply at Average Dose (July 2017)
Paliperidone palmitate (Invega Trinza) 2015	Schizophrenia (only after at least 4 months of adequate treatment on Invega Sustenna)	273, 410, 546, 819 mg in prefilled syringes	No overlap	3 months	Based on previous Invega Sustenna dose: • for 78 mg, give 273 mg Trinza • for 117 mg, give 410 mg Trinza • for 156 mg, give 546 mg Trinza • for 234 mg, give 819 mg Trinza	Give same conversion dose of Trinza every 3 months; adjust if necessary per patient response	$$$$$
Risperidone (Risperdal Consta) 2003	Schizophrenia Bipolar, manic/mixed (monotherapy or adjunct)	12.5, 25, 37.5, and 50 mg vials	With usual oral dose for 3 weeks	2 weeks	Start at 25 mg Q2 weeks. Adjust dose no more frequently than Q4 weeks as needed for response.	Approx. equivalence: <4 mg/day oral: 25 mg 4 mg–6 mg/day oral: 37.5 mg >6 mg/day oral: 50 mg Maximum dose: 50 mg Q2 weeks	$$$$$

[1]brand discontinued; available as generic only

Antipsychotics

Anxiolytic Medications

GENERAL PRESCRIBING TIPS

Although antidepressants are arguably the most effective medications for anxiety, in this chapter we focus on benzodiazepines and other drugs used specifically for anxiety disorders.

Psychiatry has long had a love/hate relationship with benzos. They work quickly and predictably, but they often lead to dependence and sometimes to outright addiction.

Assuming you've done a good enough diagnostic evaluation to identify malingerers and drug abusers, here's a reasonable approach to deciding on which anxiolytic medication to prescribe.

1. Start with a long-acting medication such as clonazepam. It's less likely to lead to addiction, because its onset and offset are more gradual.
2. Reserve short-acting benzos, like alprazolam or lorazepam, for patients who have occasional anxiety, and prescribe these on an as-needed basis.
3. When treating anxiety disorders that are responsive to antidepressants (and which ones aren't?), do the following: Start patients on an SSRI/SNRI plus a benzo. Tell them that in 2 weeks they will be able to stop taking the benzo because the antidepressant will have kicked in.
4. Give buspirone a chance, especially for generalized anxiety disorder. It may not work as reliably as benzos, but it is non-addictive.
5. Don't forget propranolol, which can be really effective for patients who have strong somatic symptoms of anxiety, such as pounding heart and shortness of breath.
6. Finally, prazosin, another blood pressure medication, is effective for PTSD, especially for insomnia and nightmares.

Class Warnings

Combining benzodiazepines with opiates

The FDA has issued a black box warning about the dangers of combining benzodiazepines with opiates due to the risks of profound sedation, respiratory depression, coma, and death. The FDA stipulates that the benzo/opioid combination should be reserved for patients when alternative options have not worked, that you should minimize the dosage and duration of treatment, and that patients should be monitored closely for sedation and respiratory depression.

Sleep architecture

Benzodiazepines affect sleep architecture; thus, long-term use is discouraged.

TABLE 8: Anxiolytic Medications

Generic Name (Brand Name) Year FDA Approved *[G] denotes generic availability*	Relevant FDA Indication(s)	Available Strengths (mg)	Onset of Action (oral)	Half-Life (hours)	Duration of Action (hours)	Usual Dosage Range (starting–max) (mg)
Alprazolam (Xanax, Xanax XR, Niravam) [G] 1981	GAD Panic disorder	Tablets: 0.25, 0.5, 1, 2 ER tablets: 0.5, 1, 2, 3 ODT: 0.25, 0.5, 1, 2 Liquid: 1 mg/mL	30 min (IR, ODT) 1–2 hrs (XR)	11–16	3–4 (IR) 10 (XR)	0.25 mg TID–2 mg TID 0.5 mg–3 mg QD (XR)
Buspirone (BuSpar[1]) [G] 1986	GAD	Tablets: 5, 7.5, 10, 15, 30	1–2 weeks+	2–3	N/A	5 mg TID–20 mg TID
Clonazepam (Klonopin, Klonopin Wafers[1]) [G] 1975	Panic disorder	Tablets: 0.5, 1, 2 ODT: 0.125, 0.25, 0.5, 1, 2	1 hr	20–80	4–8	0.5 mg BID–2 mg TID
Diazepam (Valium) [G] 1963	GAD Alcohol withdrawal	Tablets: 2, 5, 10 Liquid: 5 mg/5 mL, 5 mg/mL Injection: 5 mg/mL	30 min	>100	4–6	2 mg BID–10 mg QID
Lorazepam (Ativan) [G] 1977	GAD	Tablets: 0.5, 1, 2 Liquid: 2 mg/mL Injection: 2 mg/mL, 4 mg/mL	30–60 min	10–20	4–6	1 mg BID–5 mg BID
Prazosin (Minipress) [G] 1976	PTSD (off-label)	Capsules: 1, 2, 5	1–2 hrs	2–3	4–6	1 mg/day–10 mg/day QHS or divided BID
Propranolol (Inderal) [G] 1973	Performance anxiety (off-label)	Tablets: 10, 20, 40, 60, 80	60 min	3–6	4–6	10–40 mg PRN

[1]Brand discontinued; available as generic only

TABLE 8.1: Benzodiazepine Dosage Equivalencies

Benzodiazepine	Approximate Equivalent Dosage (mg)
Alprazolam (Xanax)	0.5
Chlordiazepoxide (Librium)	25
Clonazepam (Klonopin)	0.25–0.5
Clorazepate (Tranxene)	7.5
Diazepam (Valium)	5
Estazolam (ProSom)	1
Flurazepam (Dalmane)	15
Lorazepam (Ativan)	1
Oxazepam (Serax)	15
Quazepam (Doral)	15
Temazepam (Restoril)	15
Triazolam (Halcion)	0.25

ALPRAZOLAM (Xanax) Fact Sheet [G]

FDA Indications:

Generalized anxiety disorder (GAD); panic disorder.

Off-Label Uses:

Other anxiety disorders; insomnia; acute mania or psychosis; catatonia.

Dosage Forms:

- **Tablets (G):** 0.25, 0.5 mg, 1 mg, 2 mg.
- **ER tablets (Xanax XR, G):** 0.5 mg, 1 mg, 2 mg, 3 mg.
- **Orally disintegrating tablets (Niravam, G):** 0.25 mg, 0.5 mg, 1 mg, 2 mg.
- **Oral concentrate (G):** 1 mg/mL.

Dosage Guidance:

- GAD: Start 0.25 mg–0.5 mg TID; increase by 0.25 mg–0.5 mg/day increments every 3–4 days as needed and tolerated to max dose 4 mg/day divided TID–QID.
- Panic disorder: Start 0.5 mg TID; increase by increments of no more than 1 mg/day every 3–4 days as needed to a target dose 4 mg–6 mg/day divided TID–QID. Max dose 10 mg/day.
- For panic disorder using XR: Start 0.5 mg–1 mg QD; increase by increments of no more than 1 mg/day at intervals of 3–4 days to target dose 3 mg–6 mg QD.

Monitoring: No routine monitoring recommended unless clinical picture warrants.

Cost: $; ODT: $$

Side Effects:

- Most common: Sedation, somnolence, memory impairment, slurred speech, incoordination, dependence.
- Serious but rare: Anterograde amnesia, increased fall risk, paradoxical reaction (irritability, agitation), respiratory depression (avoid in patients with sleep apnea).

Mechanism, Pharmacokinetics, and Drug Interactions:

- Binds to benzodiazepine receptors to enhance GABA effects.
- Metabolized primarily through CYP3A4; t ½: 11–16 hours.
- Avoid use with other CNS depressants, including alcohol and opioids (additive effects). Potent CYP3A4 inhibitors (eg, fluvoxamine, erythromycin) may increase alprazolam levels; CYP3A4 inducers (eg, carbamazepine) may decrease alprazolam levels.

Clinical Pearls:

- Schedule IV controlled substance.
- Benzodiazepines are very effective immediately for GAD and panic disorder, particularly in the early weeks of SSRI therapy while awaiting onset of therapeutic effect.
- Paradoxical reaction of aggression, agitation, and combativeness is more likely to occur in the elderly or those with brain injury.
- While benzodiazepines are highly abusable, patients with panic disorder rarely self-increase their dose when treated adequately, indicating that tolerance to anxiolytic effects does not occur.

Fun Fact:

There are many slang terms for alprazolam; some of the more common ones are Bars, Z-bars, Zannies, Footballs, Blues, or Blue Footballs.

Bottom Line:

Fast-acting and effective for GAD and panic disorder, but short duration of action may contribute to breakthrough symptoms between doses and make withdrawal more difficult.

BUSPIRONE (BuSpar) Fact Sheet [G]

FDA Indications:
Generalized anxiety disorder (GAD).

Off-Label Uses:
Treatment-resistant depression; anxiety symptoms in depression.

Dosage Forms:
Tablets (G): 5 mg, 7.5 mg, 10 mg, 15 mg, 30 mg (scored).

Dosage Guidance:
Start 7.5 mg BID or 5 mg TID; increase by increments of 5 mg/day every 2–3 days to target dose 20 mg–30 mg/day divided BID–TID; max 20 mg TID.

Monitoring: No routine monitoring recommended unless clinical picture warrants.

Cost: $

Side Effects:
Most common: Dizziness, nervousness, nausea, headache, jitteriness.

Mechanism, Pharmacokinetics, and Drug Interactions:
- Serotonin 5HT1A receptor partial agonist.
- Metabolized primarily through CYP3A4; t ½: 2–3 hours.
- Avoid use with MAOIs; caution with serotonergic agents due to additive effects and risk for serotonin syndrome. Caution with 3A4 inhibitors or inducers as they may affect buspirone serum levels; adjust dose.

Clinical Pearls:
- Similar to antidepressants, buspirone requires 1–2 weeks for onset of therapeutic effects, with full effects occurring over several weeks, and offers no "as-needed" benefits.
- Non-sedating, non-habit-forming alternative to benzodiazepines for anxiety. May be less effective or ineffective in patients who have previously responded to benzos.
- Has only shown efficacy in GAD, not in other anxiety disorders (PTSD, OCD, panic disorder).
- May potentiate antidepressant effects when used in combination with SSRIs in refractory depression.

Fun Fact:
Other psychotropic agents with 5HT1A partial agonist effects include aripiprazole, ziprasidone, and vilazodone.

Bottom Line:
An alternative to benzodiazepine in patients for whom benzos are not appropriate. Don't expect as robust a response, though.

CLONAZEPAM (Klonopin) Fact Sheet [G]

FDA Indications:
Seizure disorders; panic disorder.

Off-Label Uses:
Other anxiety disorders; insomnia; acute mania or psychosis; catatonia.

Dosage Forms:
- **Tablets (G):** 0.5 mg, 1 mg, 2 mg.
- **Orally disintegrating tablets (G):** 0.125 mg, 0.25 mg, 0.5 mg, 1 mg, 2 mg.

Dosage Guidance:
- Dose varies based on patient characteristics (eg, age) and tolerance to benzodiazepines.
- Anxiety: Start 0.5 mg BID; increase by 0.5 mg–1 mg/day increments every 2–4 days to max 6 mg/day divided BID–TID.
- Insomnia (off-label use): Start 0.25 mg–0.5 mg QHS as needed for insomnia. Max 2 mg at bedtime.
- Use lower doses for elderly.

Monitoring: No routine monitoring recommended unless clinical picture warrants.

Cost: $

Side Effects:
- Most common: Somnolence, daytime grogginess, confusion, ataxia.
- Serious but rare: Anterograde amnesia, increased fall risk, paradoxical reaction (irritability, agitation), respiratory depression (avoid in patients with sleep apnea).

Mechanism, Pharmacokinetics, and Drug Interactions:
- Binds to benzodiazepine receptors to enhance GABA effects.
- Metabolized primarily through CYP3A4; t ½: 20–80 hours.
- Avoid concomitant use with other CNS depressants, including alcohol and opioids (additive effects). Potent CYP3A4 inhibitors (eg, fluvoxamine, erythromycin) may increase clonazepam levels; CYP3A4 inducers (eg, carbamazepine) may decrease clonazepam levels.

Clinical Pearls:
- Schedule IV controlled substance.
- High potency, long-acting benzodiazepine with active metabolites that may accumulate.
- Withdrawal effects may not be seen until 3–5 days after abrupt discontinuation and may last 10–14 days due to long half-life and active metabolites of clonazepam.
- Full effects of a particular dose may not be evident for a few days since active metabolites will accumulate with continual use (versus PRN use). Wait several days before increasing dose if patient is taking clonazepam regularly.

Fun Fact:
Klonopin tablets (or "K-pins") have a street value of $2–$5 per tablet, depending on dose and geographic region.

Bottom Line:
Fewer breakthrough symptoms compared to alprazolam when used for anxiety due to longer half-life. May work as a good hypnotic for the short term, although dependence and long half-life limit this use.

DIAZEPAM (Valium) Fact Sheet [G]

FDA Indications:
Generalized anxiety disorder (GAD); alcohol withdrawal; seizures; muscle spasms.

Off-Label Uses:
Other anxiety disorders; insomnia; acute mania or psychosis; catatonia.

Dosage Forms:
- **Tablets (G):** 2 mg, 5 mg, 10 mg (scored).
- **Oral liquid (G):** 5 mg/5 mL, 5 mg/1 mL.
- **Injection (G):** 5 mg/1 mL.

Dosage Guidance:
Anxiety: Start 2 mg BID–5 mg BID; increase by 2 mg–5 mg/day increments every 2–4 days to max 40 mg/day divided BID–QID.

Monitoring: No routine monitoring recommended unless clinical picture warrants.

Cost: $

Side Effects:
- Most common: Somnolence, daytime grogginess, confusion, ataxia.
- Serious but rare: Anterograde amnesia, increased fall risk, paradoxical reaction (irritability, agitation), respiratory depression (avoid in patients with sleep apnea).

Mechanism, Pharmacokinetics, and Drug Interactions:
- Binds to benzodiazepine receptors to enhance GABA effects.
- Metabolized primarily through CYP3A4 and 2C19; t ½: >100 hours.
- Avoid concomitant use with other CNS depressants, including alcohol and opioids (additive effects).

Clinical Pearls:
- Schedule IV controlled substance.
- Long-acting benzodiazepine with active metabolites that may accumulate.
- Tolerance to sedative effect may develop more rapidly (within 2–4 weeks of use) than tolerance to anti-anxiety effect.
- Withdrawal effects may not be seen until 3–5 days after abrupt discontinuation and may last 10–14 days due to long half-life and active metabolites of diazepam.
- Diazepam has the highest lipid solubility of all benzos, which means very rapid distribution into and out of the CNS, resulting in the greatest "rush" felt by patients using in a single-dose manner. This feature makes diazepam the most abusable benzo.

Fun Fact:
Valium has been glorified in music more than once. The Rolling Stones' "little yellow pill" in "Mother's Little Helper" and Lou Reed's "Walk on the Wild Side" ("Jackie is just speeding away/Thought she was James Dean for a day/Then I guess she had to crash/Valium would have helped that bash") are two good examples.

Bottom Line:
Diazepam has a long history of use with good efficacy for anxiety. Its long half-life makes it a particularly effective anxiolytic for some patients.

LORAZEPAM (Ativan) Fact Sheet [G]

FDA Indications:

Generalized anxiety disorder (GAD); status epilepticus (IV route).

Off-Label Uses:

Other anxiety disorders; insomnia; acute mania or psychosis; catatonia.

Dosage Forms:

- **Tablets (G):** 0.5 mg, 1 mg, 2 mg.
- **Oral concentrate (G):** 2 mg/mL.
- **Injection (G):** 2 mg/mL, 4 mg/mL.

Dosage Guidance:

- Anxiety: Start 1 mg BID; increase by 0.5 mg–1 mg/day increments every 2–4 days up to 6 mg/day divided BID–TID. Max 10 mg/day divided BID–TID.
- Insomnia (off-label use): Start 0.5 mg–1 mg QHS, 20–30 minutes before bedtime; max 4 mg nightly.
- Use lower doses in elderly.

Monitoring: No routine monitoring recommended unless clinical picture warrants.

Cost: $

Side Effects:

- Most common: Somnolence, dizziness, weakness, ataxia.
- Serious but rare: Anterograde amnesia, increased fall risk, paradoxical reaction (irritability, agitation), respiratory depression (avoid in patients with sleep apnea).

Mechanism, Pharmacokinetics, and Drug Interactions:

- Binds to benzodiazepine receptors to enhance GABA effects.
- Metabolism primarily hepatic (non-CYP450) to inactive compounds; t ½: 10–20 hours.
- Avoid concomitant use with other CNS depressants, including alcohol and opioids (additive effects). No risk for CYP450 drug interactions.

Clinical Pearls:

- Schedule IV controlled substance.
- Lorazepam does not have a long half-life or active metabolites that could accumulate, and poses no CYP450 drug interaction risk.
- Withdrawal symptoms usually seen on the first day after abrupt discontinuation and last 5–7 days in patients receiving short–intermediate half-life benzodiazepines such as lorazepam. A gradual taper is highly recommended, particularly if the patient is receiving prolonged treatment on a high dose.
- Tolerance to sedative effect may develop within 2–4 weeks of use, and benzodiazepines affect sleep architecture; thus, long-term use is discouraged.

Fun Fact:

Early Ativan marketing efforts included clever direct-to-consumer advertising campaigns. These included "Now it can be yours—The Ativan experience" in 1977 and "In a world where certainties are few . . . no wonder Ativan is prescribed by so many caring clinicians" in 1987.

Bottom Line:

When a benzodiazepine is appropriate for use (short-term; minimal risk of abuse), we consider lorazepam to be a first-line agent.

PRAZOSIN (Minipress) Fact Sheet [G]

FDA Indications:
Hypertension.

Off-Label Uses:
PTSD.

Dosage Forms:
Capsules (G): 1 mg, 2 mg, 5 mg.

Dosage Guidance:
- PTSD (off-label): Titrate dose slowly to minimize possibility of "first-dose" orthostatic hypotension. Start 1 mg QHS x 3 days, then 2 mg QHS x 4 days. If tolerating but still symptomatic, increase to 3 mg QHS x 7 days. Dose can be increased further, based on response, to 4 mg QHS x 7 days. Target 1 mg–5 mg/day.
- May dose-divide BID to target daytime PTSD-associated arousal symptoms.

Monitoring: Periodic blood pressure.

Cost: $

Side Effects:
- Most common: Somnolence, dizziness, headache, weakness.
- Serious but rare: Orthostasis and syncope; prolonged erections and priapism have been reported.

Mechanism, Pharmacokinetics, and Drug Interactions:
- Alpha-1 adrenergic receptor antagonist.
- Metabolism primarily hepatic (non-CYP450); t ½: 2–3 hours.
- Caution with other antihypertensive agents, diuretics, and PDE5 inhibitors (eg, Viagra) that may have additive hypotensive effects.

Clinical Pearls:
Initial studies showed improvement in trauma-related nightmares and sleep quality when dosed at bedtime as well as positive effects on daytime PTSD symptoms when dosed BID. However, a subsequent and more recent study in veterans found it no better than placebo.

Fun Fact:
Prazosin is an older drug, which is now rarely used for its original indication (hypertension). It's now used as a second-line agent for urinary hesitancy in benign prostatic hyperplasia. It is also being investigated for alcohol dependence.

Bottom Line:
Though the evidence is mixed, consider a trial of prazosin for PTSD in some of your patients, especially for those with PTSD-associated nightmares.

PROPRANOLOL (Inderal) Fact Sheet [G]

FDA Indications:
Hypertension; angina; post-MI cardioprotection; atrial fibrillation; migraine prophylaxis; essential tremor.

Off-Label Uses:
Performance anxiety, tremor due to medication side effects (especially lithium).

Dosage Forms:
Tablets (G): 10 mg, 20 mg, 40 mg, 60 mg, 80 mg (scored).

Dosage Guidance:
- Performance anxiety (off-label use): Give 10 mg about 60 minutes prior to performance; usual effective dose is 10 mg–40 mg.
- Medication-induced tremor: Start 10 mg BID as needed; can go up to 30 mg–120 mg daily in two or three divided doses. Can also use Inderal LA, long-acting version of propranolol, 60 mg–80 mg once a day.

Monitoring: Periodic blood pressure/pulse.

Cost: $

Side Effects:
Most common: Dizziness, fatigue, bradycardia, and hypotension.

Mechanism, Pharmacokinetics, and Drug Interactions:
- Non-selective beta-1 and beta-2 adrenergic receptor antagonist.
- Metabolized primarily through CYP2D6, also 1A2 and 2C19; t ½: 3–6 hours.
- Caution with other antihypertensives (additive effects). CYP2D6 inhibitors, as well as inhibitors or inducers of 1A2 and 2C19, may affect propranolol levels.

Clinical Pearl:
With beta blockade, propranolol reduces some of the somatic symptoms of anxiety (tremor, sweating, flushing, tachycardia).

Fun Fact:
The list of notable people who suffer or have suffered from performance anxiety or stage fright is long. It includes Barbra Streisand, Carly Simon, Van Morrison, Frédéric Chopin, Renee Fleming, Jay Mohr, Hugh Grant, Laurence Olivier, Mahatma Gandhi, and Thomas Jefferson, among others.

Bottom Line:
Effective and safe for use in performance anxiety, particularly when the sedating or cognitive side effects of benzos could interfere with an individual's performance.

Dementia Medications

GENERAL PRESCRIBING TIPS

While it's good that we have a handful of FDA-approved drugs for dementia, the fact is that they do not work very well. In clinical settings, it is usually impossible to know whether they are working at all. This is because they work by slowing the inexorable cognitive decline seen in dementia. It is important to explain this point to family members, who might otherwise expect to see actual improvement in cognition, which is unusual. Nonetheless, starting medication close to the onset of symptoms and adjusting the dose or combining agents from different classes can reduce cognitive and functional decline as well as delay nursing home admission.

For mild to moderate dementia, start with one of the 3 approved cholinesterase inhibitors (CI). These include donepezil, galantamine, and rivastigmine. Start with donepezil (we have the most data and experience with this agent, though the others are equally effective). Titrate donepezil to an effective dose, which is 5 mg–10 mg a day (Deardorff WJ et al, *Drugs Aging* 2015;32:537–547).

For moderate to severe Alzheimer's dementia, for an FDA-approved approach, you can start with either memantine IR or high-dose donepezil (either by combining two 10 mgs or using the 23 mg version). Reserve the more expensive memantine XR for those rare situations in which IR is poorly tolerated.

An alternative approach is to follow the same protocol for all your patients with dementia, whether or not it is "severe" or "moderate." Start with a combination of donepezil and memantine, and for patients who have trouble taking two pills, consider Namzaric, which is the combination donepezil/memantine.

All 3 CIs commonly cause nausea, vomiting, and dizziness, and this is why the recommended dosing schedule is excruciatingly slow, generally no faster than 1 increment every 4 weeks. How long should patients be treated with these agents? If they are tolerated, a case can be made that you should never stop them. We say this because very long-term studies have shown that discontinuing donepezil after 6 months causes patients' cognitive scores to plummet to the level of placebo-treated patients. And even when these patients were "rescued" with donepezil, cognitive decline continued. So if a patient has tolerated a CI for several months, keep the prescription going indefinitely.

TABLE 9: Dementia Medications

Generic Name (Brand Name) Year FDA Approved *[G] denotes generic availability*	Relevant FDA Indication(s)	Available Strengths (mg except where noted)	Usual Dosage Range (starting–max) (mg)
Donepezil (Aricept, Aricept ODT) [G] 1996	Mild to moderate Alzheimer's dementia (5, 10 mg) Moderate to severe Alzheimer's dementia (10, 23 mg)	Tablets: 5, 10, 23 ODT: 5, 10	5 QAM–23 QAM
Galantamine (Razadyne) [G] 2001	Mild to moderate Alzheimer's dementia	Tablets: 4, 8, 12 Liquid: 4 mg/mL	4 BID–12 BID
Galantamine ER (Razadyne ER) [G] 2004	Mild to moderate Alzheimer's dementia	ER capsules: 8, 16, 24	8 ER QAM–24 ER QAM
Memantine (Namenda) [G] 2003	Moderate to severe Alzheimer's dementia	Tablets: 5, 10 Liquid: 10 mg/5 mL	5 QAM–10 BID
Memantine ER (Namenda XR) 2010	Moderate to severe Alzheimer's dementia	ER capsules: 7, 14, 21, 28	7–28 QD
Memantine ER/donepezil (Namzaric) 2014	Moderate to severe Alzheimer's dementia (in patients already stabilized on both medications)	ER capsules: 7/10, 14/10, 21/10, 28/10	Patients on memantine (10 mg BID or 28 mg XR QD) and donepezil 10 mg QD can be switched to Namzaric 28 mg/10 mg QPM
Rivastigmine (Exelon) [G] 2000	Mild to moderate Alzheimer's dementia Mild to moderate dementia associated with Parkinson's disease	Capsules: 1.5, 3, 4.5, 6	1.5 BID–6 BID
Rivastigmine (Exelon Patch) [G] 2007	Mild to moderate and severe Alzheimer's dementia Mild to moderate dementia associated with Parkinson's disease	ER patches: 4.6, 9.5, 13.3/24 hr	4.6 mg/24 hr QD–13.3 mg/24 hr QD

DONEPEZIL (Aricept) Fact Sheet [G]

FDA Indications:

Mild to moderate Alzheimer's dementia (5 mg, 10 mg); **moderate to severe Alzheimer's dementia** (10 mg, 23 mg).

Off-Label Uses:

Other memory disorders; mild cognitive impairment.

Dosage Forms:

- **Tablets (G):** 5 mg, 10 mg, 23 mg.
- **Orally disintegrating tablets (Aricept ODT, G):** 5 mg, 10 mg.

Dosage Guidance:

- Mild to moderate dementia: Start 5 mg QD and ↑ to 10 mg QD after 4–6 weeks.
- Moderate to severe dementia: May ↑ further to 23 mg QD after ≥3 months (range 10 mg–23 mg/day).

Monitoring: No routine monitoring recommended unless clinical picture warrants.

Cost: 5 mg, 10 mg: $; 23 mg: $$

Side Effects:

- Most common: Dose-related diarrhea, nausea, vomiting, weight loss (especially 23 mg/day dose), anorexia, insomnia, abnormal dreams.
- Serious but rare: Cholinesterase inhibitors may have vagotonic effects that may cause bradycardia and/or heart block with or without a history of cardiac disease; syncope reported.

Mechanism, Pharmacokinetics, and Drug Interactions:

- Acetylcholinesterase (AChE) inhibitor.
- Metabolized primarily through CYP2D6 and 3A4; t ½: 70 hours.
- Avoid use with anticholinergic agents as they will diminish therapeutic effects; avoid beta blockers due to risk of bradycardia. P450 interactions not usually clinically important.

Clinical Pearls:

- Donepezil is the second drug to be approved for dementia after tacrine, which was pulled from the market due to liver toxicity; donepezil is also the most prescribed of the 3 CIs. It received additional FDA approval for use in severe dementia (in addition to its initial approval for mild to moderate dementia).
- The manufacturer recommends bedtime dosing, but giving it in the morning may prevent the insomnia and vivid dreams some patients report with donepezil.
- Once-a-day dosing and easy titration makes this agent simplest to use.
- GI side effects usually resolve in 1–2 weeks.
- Based on a Cochrane review, donepezil causes fewer side effects than rivastigmine.
- Be mindful of other medications that may have intrinsic anticholinergic activity; these will counteract donepezil's therapeutic effects.

Fun Fact:

Donepezil has been studied in children for autism, pervasive developmental disorders, ADHD, and tic disorders; however, the minimal data do not support such use.

Bottom Line:

First-line agent, but don't expect big improvements.

GALANTAMINE (Razadyne) Fact Sheet [G]

FDA Indications:
Mild to moderate Alzheimer's dementia.

Off-Label Uses:
Other memory disorders; mild cognitive impairment.

Dosage Forms:
- **Tablets (G):** 4 mg, 8 mg, 12 mg.
- **ER capsules (Razadyne ER, G):** 8 mg, 16 mg, 24 mg.
- **Oral solution:** 4 mg/mL.

Dosage Guidance:
- IR: Start 4 mg BID (breakfast and dinner), ↑ by 4 mg BID increments every 4 weeks.
- ER: Start 8 mg QAM (breakfast), ↑ by 8 mg/day every 4 weeks.
- For both, max 24 mg/day (target dose: 16 mg–24 mg/day).
- If using oral solution, mix dose with 3–4 ounces of any nonalcoholic beverage; mix well and drink immediately.
- If therapy is interrupted for ≥3 days, restart at the lowest dose and increase to current dose.

Monitoring: No routine monitoring recommended unless clinical picture warrants.

Cost: $$; liquid: $$$$

Side Effects:
- Most common: Diarrhea, nausea, vomiting, weight loss, anorexia, insomnia, abnormal dreams.
- Serious but rare: Cholinesterase inhibitors may have vagotonic effects that may cause bradycardia and/or heart block with or without a history of cardiac disease; syncope reported.

Mechanism, Pharmacokinetics, and Drug Interactions:
- Acetylcholinesterase (AChE) inhibitor and cholinergic nicotinic receptor modulator.
- Metabolized primarily through CYP2D6 and 3A4; t ½: 7 hours.
- Avoid use with anticholinergic agents as they will diminish therapeutic effects; avoid beta blockers due to risk of bradycardia. P450 interactions not usually clinically important.

Clinical Pearls:
- Galantamine's claim to fame is that it has a "dual" mechanism of action, modulating cholinergic nicotinic receptors in addition to inhibiting AChE. The manufacturer may use this factoid to argue that galantamine is more effective than the other CIs. However, accumulating evidence seems to show no difference in efficacy (Birks J. Cholinesterase inhibitors for Alzheimer's disease. *Cochrane Database Syst Rev* 2006).
- ER formulation seems to be used more often due to ease of once-daily dosing.

Fun Fact:
Razadyne was approved in 2001 with its original name, Reminyl. Pharmacists were sometimes confusing written scripts for Reminyl with Amaryl, a diabetes medication. In April 2005, the trade name was changed to Razadyne to avoid future dispensing errors.

Bottom Line:
No appreciable benefit over donepezil, which has spent a longer time on the market and has a greater range of experience given additional indication for severe dementia; consider this a second-line agent.

MEMANTINE (Namenda) Fact Sheet [G]

FDA Indications:
Moderate to severe Alzheimer's dementia.

Off-Label Uses:
Mild to moderate Alzheimer's dementia; other memory disorders; mild cognitive impairment; chronic pain.

Dosage Forms:
- **Tablets (G):** 5 mg, 10 mg.
- **Oral solution (G):** 10 mg/5 mL.
- **ER capsules (Namenda XR):** 7 mg, 14 mg, 21 mg, 28 mg.

Dosage Guidance:
- IR: 5 mg QD week 1; 5 mg BID week 2; 10 mg QAM and 5 mg QHS week 3; 10 mg BID week 4 and beyond.
- XR: Start 7 mg QD; ↑ by 7 mg/day in increments ≥1 week to max dose 28 mg/day (10 mg BID equivalent to 28 mg XR QD). Can be opened and sprinkled on food.

Monitoring: No routine monitoring recommended unless clinical picture warrants.

Cost: IR: $; ER, liquid: $$$$

Side Effects:
Most common: Dizziness (XR), transient confusion (IR), headache (XR), diarrhea (XR), constipation, sedation.

Mechanism, Pharmacokinetics, and Drug Interactions:
- N-methyl-D-aspartate (NMDA) receptor antagonist.
- Metabolism primarily hepatic, but not P450; t ½: 60–80 hours.
- Pharmacokinetic interactions unlikely.

Clinical Pearls:
- FDA-approved for moderate to severe Alzheimer's dementia only; may also be effective as augmentation added to donepezil in patients with moderate to severe Alzheimer's dementia (see memantine ER/donepezil fact sheet).
- Data comparing 10 mg BID and 20 mg QD of IR formulation, as well as pharmacokinetic profile, support use of once-daily IR dosing; IR is used QD in Europe.

Fun Fact:
Forest Pharmaceuticals had announced it was discontinuing sales of the IR formulation as of August 15, 2014, in order to "focus on" the XR formulation—just ahead of the IR patent expiration. However, the New York attorney general filed an antitrust lawsuit, claiming this was an anticompetitive move, and Forest was forced to continue offering both Namenda IR and Namenda XR.

Bottom Line:
Memantine's indication (moderate to severe dementia only) may limit its use, but it does boast a unique mechanism of action and has some data to support its usefulness as an augmenter of donepezil. Many prescribers put the majority of their dementia patients on a combination of one of the CIs and memantine; we recommend adding memantine when dementia has progressed to the moderate or severe level, possibly earlier. There's no clinical benefit to using the more expensive XR version.

MEMANTINE ER/DONEPEZIL (Namzaric) Fact Sheet

FDA Indications:
Moderate to severe Alzheimer's dementia.

Off-Label Uses:
Mild to moderate Alzheimer's dementia; other memory disorders; mild cognitive impairment.

Dosage Forms:
Capsules: 7 mg/10 mg, 14 mg/10 mg, 21 mg/10 mg, 28 mg/10 mg memantine ER and donepezil.

Dosage Guidance:
- Patients should first be stabilized on the individual medications; patients on memantine (10 mg BID or 28 mg XR QD) and donepezil 10 mg QD can be switched to Namzaric 28 mg/10 mg QPM.
- Patients with severe renal impairment on memantine 5 mg BID or 14 mg XR QD and donepezil 10 mg QD can be switched to Namzaric 14 mg/10 mg QPM.

Monitoring: No routine monitoring recommended unless clinical picture warrants.

Cost: $$$$

Side Effects:
- Most common: Headache, diarrhea, dizziness, vomiting, weight loss, anorexia, insomnia, abnormal dreams.
- Serious but rare: Cholinesterase inhibitors may have vagotonic effects that may cause bradycardia and/or heart block with or without a history of cardiac disease; syncope reported.

Mechanism, Pharmacokinetics, and Drug Interactions:
- N-methyl-D-aspartate (NMDA) receptor antagonist and acetylcholinesterase (AChE) inhibitor.
- Metabolism: Memantine hepatic but not P450, and donepezil primarily through CYP2D6 and 3A4; t ½: 60–80 hours (memantine) and 70 hours (donepezil).
- Avoid use with anticholinergic agents as they will diminish therapeutic effects; avoid beta blockers due to risk of bradycardia. P450 interactions not usually clinically important.

Clinical Pearls:
- Many experts now stabilize patients on an AChE inhibitor like donepezil and then add memantine.
- The manufacturer recommends bedtime dosing, but taking it in the morning may prevent the insomnia and vivid dreams some patients report with donepezil.
- Once-a-day dosing makes this agent easiest to use.
- Be mindful of other medications that may have intrinsic anticholinergic activity; these will counteract donepezil's therapeutic effects.

Fun Fact:
In 2014, Actavis Pharmaceuticals acquired Forest Pharmaceuticals, manufacturer of Namzaric. That same year, Actavis also acquired Allergan, manufacturer of Botox, another medication targeting the aging process but in a different way.

Bottom Line:
For patients who are already on this regimen but have trouble taking two pills, consider Namzaric.

RIVASTIGMINE (Exelon, Exelon Patch) Fact Sheet [G]

FDA Indications:

Mild to moderate Alzheimer's dementia (capsules); **mild to moderate and severe Alzheimer's dementia** (patch); **dementia associated with Parkinson's disease** (capsules and patch).

Off-Label Uses:

Other memory disorders; mild cognitive impairment.

Dosage Forms:

- **Capsules (G):** 1.5 mg, 3 mg, 4.5 mg, 6 mg.
- **Transdermal patches (G):** 4.6 mg/24 hour, 9.5 mg/24 hour, 13.3 mg/24 hour, containing rivastigmine 9 mg, 18 mg, and 27 mg, respectively.

Dosage Guidance:

- Start 1.5 mg BID with meals for 4 weeks, ↑ by 1.5 mg BID increments every 4 weeks, up to max 6 mg BID with meals.
- Patch: For mild to moderate dementia, start 4.6 mg/24 hours; if tolerated, ↑ after ≥4 weeks to 9.5 mg/24 hours (target and max dose). For severe dementia, titrate to 13.3 mg/24 hour (effective and max dose).
- Converting oral to patch: <6 mg/day: Use 4.6 mg/24 hour patch; 6 mg–12 mg/day: Use 9.5 mg/24 hour patch; apply patch on next day following last oral dose.

Monitoring: No routine monitoring recommended unless clinical picture warrants.

Cost: Oral: $$; patch: $$$

Side Effects:

- Most common: Dizziness, headache, diarrhea, anorexia, nausea, vomiting, skin reactions (patch).
- Serious but rare: Cholinesterase inhibitors may have vagotonic effects that may cause bradycardia and/or heart block with or without a history of cardiac disease; syncope reported.

Mechanism, Pharmacokinetics, and Drug Interactions:

- Acetylcholinesterase (AChE) and butyrylcholinesterase (BuChE) inhibitor.
- Metabolized extensively, although CYP enzymes minimally involved; t ½: 1.5 hours (oral); 3 hours (after patch removal).
- Avoid use with anticholinergic agents as they will diminish therapeutic effects; avoid beta blockers due to risk of bradycardia. P450 interactions not likely.

Clinical Pearls:

- Only CI with additional indication for Parkinson's-related dementia.
- Rivastigmine inhibits both AChE and the nonspecific BuChE (also known as pseudocholinesterase), which is mostly found in the liver and GI tract; this may explain why rivastigmine causes significant GI side effects.
- Rivastigmine transdermal patches may cause less nausea and vomiting.

Fun Fact:

Exelon is also the name of a corporation that provides energy services (electric and natural gas) and is the largest nuclear operator in the United States.

Bottom Line:

Since all CIs are equally effective, we recommend starting with donepezil, which offers once-daily dosing, generic availability, and a good tolerability profile. Rivastigmine remains second-line due to BID dosing, cost, and unacceptably high rates of nausea and vomiting.

Hypnotics

GENERAL PRESCRIBING TIPS

The major challenge in prescribing hypnotics is finding something that works but that does not cause long-term dependence. The best way to achieve this goal is to avoid prescribing benzodiazepines as sleeping pills.

The preferred way to treat insomnia is to treat the underlying cause, which in most of our patients is usually either a psychiatric disorder or a side effect of a medication for that disorder. A common scenario is the patient who presents with major depression with insomnia as one of the depressive symptoms. In this case, either prescribe an antidepressant alone, or an antidepressant plus a 2-week prescription for a hypnotic. In most cases, the antidepressant will have kicked in around the 2-week point, and your patient will no longer need the hypnotic.

If treating the underlying condition doesn't work, you should discuss sleep hygiene techniques, though in our experience these don't do the trick for most psychiatric patients. Although cognitive behavior therapy for chronic insomnia can be effective, it is challenging to find a local therapist who is skilled in the techniques involved.

Once you and your patient have resigned yourselves to a hypnotic, there's a pretty long menu of reasonable offerings. The choices below are not listed in any particular order, because we don't really have any specific recommendations one way or another. We tend to pick and choose among them, which often requires trials of more than one before hitting on the sleep ambrosia for a particular patient.

- **"Z-drugs"** (eszopiclone, zaleplon, zolpidem) bind selectively to specific subunits of the GABA receptors that induce sleep, but they don't have the same relaxation effects of benzos and are probably somewhat less addictive. Zolpidem 5 mg–10 mg has become an old standard. For patients who wake up in the middle of the night, use zaleplon instead, because of its very short duration of action.
- **Antihistamines** (diphenhydramine and doxylamine) are over-the-counter agents that induce sedation by blocking histamine H1 receptors. Start with diphenhydramine 25 mg QHS and increase to 50 mg if needed. The older the patient, the less appropriate this option, as antihistamines can cause confusion when used chronically. While this can occur with anyone, it's more common in the elderly.
- **Benzodiazepines.** While we are aware of the dangers of tolerance, some patients take 0.5 mg of one of the benzos every night and seem to suffer no ill effects, and there is often no dosage creep over many years or even decades.
- **Ramelteon** is a melatonin agonist.
- **Suvorexant** is in a new class of agents called **dual orexin (OX1 and OX2) receptor antagonists,** or DORAs for short.
- **Doxepin** (Silenor) was approved by the FDA for use as a hypnotic. It is an old drug in new clothing—a tricyclic antidepressant being used for its antihistamine properties. Because it is expensive, we suggest using a low dose of generic doxepin to achieve the same effects as Silenor. This may entail prescribing the liquid version in order to get to doses in the 3 mg range.
- **Trazodone,** another antidepressant, is commonly used for insomnia at a dose of 25 mg–50 mg QHS. You can find the fact sheet for trazodone in the Antidepressants chapter.

Potential Side Effects of Most Hypnotics

Although taken by millions, hypnotics are a high-risk class of medications, especially for the elderly, who are at greater risk for confusion, memory problems, and gait disturbances (sometimes leading to falls). Therefore, try to avoid hypnotics in the elderly, and when you do use them, use the lowest effective dose for the shortest duration of time possible.

Certain precautions apply to most hypnotics, and we'll list them below to minimize repetition in the fact sheets:

- **Daytime grogginess or hangover effect:** Most likely to occur with antihistamines or with longer-acting benzodiazepines or extended release zolpidem.
- **Anterograde amnesia:** Most likely to occur with benzodiazepines and Z-drugs. Among benzos, triazolam (Halcion) has a particularly bad rep. Just avoid triazolam—there's no need to prescribe it given the wealth of alternatives.
- **CNS depression:** Hypnotics may impair physical or mental abilities and alertness; advise patients to use caution when performing tasks that require alertness (eg, driving).

- **Respiratory depression:** Benzodiazepines in particular may depress respiration; avoid in patients at risk, including those with COPD or sleep apnea, or those taking other depressants such as opiates. In fact, the FDA issued a black box warning about the dangers of combining benzodiazepines with opiates due to a concerning incidence of serious side effects with the combination, including profound sedation, respiratory depression, coma, and death (see the Anxiolytics chapter introduction for more details on this warning).
- **Paradoxical reactions,** including hyperactive or aggressive behavior, have been reported, and are particularly seen with benzodiazepines; younger patients, elderly, and those with head injury or organic brain syndromes are at greatest risk.
- **Tolerance** to sedating effects of benzodiazepines generally occurs after several weeks of continuous use (one-third of patients will experience tolerance after 4 weeks of use). Tolerance to anxiolytic effects occurs more slowly, and to anti-seizure effects very little or not at all. Psychological and physical dependence occurs with prolonged use.
- **Discontinuation syndrome:** Withdrawal effects occur with most hypnotics and include rebound insomnia, agitation, anxiety, and malaise. Discontinuation syndromes from benzodiazepines are most severe with longer-term use, higher doses, and shorter-acting agents; in severe cases, discontinuation may include seizures. Hypnotics should not be abruptly discontinued; doses should be tapered gradually.
- **Recreational use and abuse** may occur with many hypnotics, particularly the benzodiazepines. Avoid or minimize use in patients who have addiction risk or when abuse is suspected.
- **Complex sleep-related behaviors** such as sleep-driving, sleep-eating, sleep-texting, and sleep-sex have been reported. Although this can occur when using benzodiazepines or Z-drugs alone and at usual therapeutic doses, they often occur with high-dose use or in combination with other CNS depressants, including alcohol. Typically, these events occur when the individual is not fully awake, and often there will be no memory of the behavior.

TABLE 10: Hypnotics

Generic Name (Brand Name) Year FDA Approved *[G] denotes generic availability*	Relevant FDA Indication(s)	Available Strengths (mg except where noted)	Usual Dosage Range for Insomnia (starting–max) (mg at HS)[1]	Onset of Action[2]	Half-Life (hours)	Duration of Action (hours)[2]
Clonazepam [G] (Klonopin, Klonopin Wafers[3]) 1975	Panic disorder Insomnia (off-label use)	Tablet: 0.5, 1, 2 ODT: 0.125, 0.25, 0.5, 1, 2	0.25 to 1	1 hr	20–80	4–8
Diphenhydramine [G] (Benadryl, others) 1946 Available OTC and Rx	Insomnia (adults and children 12+ years)	Capsule: 25, 50 Liquid: 12.5 mg/mL	25–50	1 hr	3.5–9	4–6
Doxepin [G] (Silenor) 2010/1969 Generic not available in 3 mg, 6 mg	Insomnia (sleep maintenance)	Tablet: 3, 6 Capsules: 10, 25, 50, 75, 100, 150 Liquid: 10 mg/mL	6	1 hr	15	4–6
Doxylamine [G] (Unisom, others) 1978 Available OTC and Rx	Nighttime sleep aid	Tablet: 25	25–50	1 hr	10	4–6
Eszopiclone [G] (Lunesta) 2004	Insomnia (sleep onset and sleep maintenance)	Tablet: 1, 2, 3	1–3	30 min	6	6–8
Flurazepam [G] (Dalmane[3]) 1970	Insomnia (short-term)	Capsule: 15, 30	15–30	30–60 min	40–100	7–8
Lorazepam [G] (Ativan) 1977	GAD Insomnia (off-label use)	Tablet: 0.5, 1, 2 Liquid: 2 mg/mL	1–4	30–60 min	10–20	4–6
Ramelteon (Rozerem) 2005	Insomnia (sleep onset)	Tablet: 8	8	30 min	1–2.6	Unknown
Suvorexant (Belsomra) 2014	Insomnia (sleep onset and sleep maintenance)	Tablet: 5, 10, 15, 20	10–20	30–60 min	12	6–8
Temazepam [G] (Restoril) 1981	Insomnia (short-term)	Capsule: 7.5, 15, 22.5, 30	15–30	30–60 min	9–18	4–6
Trazodone [G] (Desyrel[3], Oleptro[3]) 1981/2010	Depression Insomnia (off-label use)	Tablet: 50, 100, 150, 300 ER tablet: 150, 300	25 to 50–200	1 hr	7–10	Unknown
Triazolam [G] (Halcion) 1982	Insomnia (short-term)	Tablet: 0.125, 0.25	0.25–0.5	15–30 min	1.5–5.5	Unknown

[1]For approximate benzodiazepine dose equivalencies, refer to Table 8.1

[2]Onset and duration vary from person to person, dose to dose, and preparation to preparation

[3]Brand discontinued; available as generic only

Generic Name (Brand Name) Year FDA Approved *[G] denotes generic availability*	Relevant FDA Indication(s)	Available Strengths (mg except where noted)	Usual Dosage Range for Insomnia (starting–max) (mg at HS)[1]	Onset of Action[2]	Half-Life (hours)	Duration of Action (hours)[2]
Zaleplon [G] (Sonata) 1999	Insomnia (short-term, sleep onset)	Capsule: 5, 10	10–20	30 min	1	4
Zolpidem [G] (Ambien, Ambien CR, Edluar, Zolpimist) 1992 Generic not available for Zolpimist or Edluar SL	Insomnia (IR: short-term, sleep onset; CR: sleep onset and maintenance)	Tablet: 5, 10 ER tablet: 6.25, 12.5 SL tablet: 5, 10 Oral spray: 5 mg/spray	10, 12.5 CR (5, 6.25 in women)	30 min	2.5–3	6–8
Zolpidem low dose (Intermezzo) [G] 2011	Difficulty falling asleep after middle-of-the-night awakening	SL tablet: 1.75, 3.5	1.75 women; 3.5 men	30 min	2.5	4

[1]For approximate benzodiazepine dose equivalencies, refer to Table 8.1

[2]Onset and duration vary from person to person, dose to dose, and preparation to preparation

[3]Brand discontinued; available as generic only

ANTIHISTAMINES (Diphenhydramine, Doxylamine) Fact Sheet [G]

FDA Indications:
Insomnia (adults, children 12–17 years); allergies; motion sickness; **antiparkinsonism**.

Off-Label Uses:
EPS; nausea and vomiting (morning sickness).

Dosage Forms:
- **Tablets, chewable tablets, caplets, capsules, and oral solutions, varies by brand:** 25 mg, 50 mg.
- **Common brand names:**
  - **Diphenhydramine:** Benadryl, Compoz, Nytol, Simply Sleep, Sleep-Eze, Sominex, Unisom SleepGels, Unisom SleepMelts, and generic.
  - **Doxylamine:** NyQuil, Unisom SleepTabs, and generic.

Dosage Guidance:
Insomnia: Start 25 mg, 30 minutes before bedtime. The dose required to induce sleep can be as low as 6.25 mg, but usual dose is 25 mg. Some patients may require 50 mg at bedtime.

Monitoring: No routine monitoring recommended unless clinical picture warrants.

Cost: $

Side Effects:
- Most common: Dry mouth, ataxia, urinary retention, constipation, drowsiness, memory problems.
- Serious but rare: Blurred vision, tachycardia.

Mechanism, Pharmacokinetics, and Drug Interactions:
- Histamine H1 antagonist.
- Metabolized by liver, primarily CYP2D6; t ½: for diphenhydramine, 3.5–9 hours; for doxylamine, 10 hours (12–15 in elderly).
- Avoid use with other antihistamines or anticholinergics (additive effects).

Clinical Pearls:
- These antihistamines non-selectively antagonize central and peripheral histamine H1 receptors. They also have secondary anticholinergic effects, which can cause side effects including dry mouth and urinary retention, as well as cognitive impairment in susceptible populations.
- Be aware that anticholinergic drugs are often used to treat or prevent extrapyramidal symptoms in patients taking antipsychotics; diphenhydramine is often chosen and dosed at night to take advantage of its sedative effect.

Fun Fact:
The name NyQuil is a portmanteau of "night" and "tranquil."

Bottom Line:
Antihistamines can be very effective sleep aids for many patients, although some patients may experience too much grogginess ("hangover") in the morning. Good first-line agents due to low risk of drug tolerance, dependence, or abuse, but exercise caution in the elderly, who may not tolerate peripheral effects.

DOXEPIN (Silenor) Fact Sheet [G]

FDA Indications:
Insomnia (sleep maintenance). Generic doxepin (at higher doses) approved for **depression, anxiety disorders**.

Off-Label Uses:
Headache; neuropathic pain; fibromyalgia; anxiety disorders.

Dosage Forms:
- **Tablets (Silenor):** 3 mg, 6 mg.
- **Capsules (G):** 10 mg, 25 mg, 50 mg, 75 mg, 100 mg, 150 mg.
- **Oral concentrate (G):** 10 mg/mL.

Dosage Guidance:
Insomnia:
- Silenor: Start 6 mg QHS (this is the starting, target, and max dose), taken within 30 minutes of bedtime. Use 3 mg/day in elderly. Avoid meals within 3 hours of taking Silenor.
- Doxepin: Start 10 mg capsule, or achieve a lower dose by using the oral concentrate or by opening the 10 mg capsule, dissolving it in a cup of juice, and drinking a portion of the juice.

Monitoring: No routine monitoring recommended unless clinical picture warrants.

Cost: Generic: $; Silenor: $$$$

Side Effects:
- Most common: Somnolence, nausea, dry mouth, constipation.
- Serious but rare: Orthostasis (more likely at higher doses).

Mechanism, Pharmacokinetics, and Drug Interactions:
- Tricyclic antidepressant with norepinephrine and serotonin reuptake inhibition and histamine H1 antagonism.
- Metabolized primarily through CYP2C19 and 2D6 (also 1A2 and 2C9 to lesser extent); t ½: 15 hours.
- Clinically significant drug interactions not likely at the low doses used for hypnotic effects.

Clinical Pearls:
- Silenor is a branded version of generic doxepin, but available in lower doses.
- Taking within 3 hours of eating delays therapeutic effect by up to 3 hours. For faster onset and to minimize next-day effects, don't take within 3 hours of a meal.

Fun Fact:
Somaxon Pharmaceuticals, the original but fledgling manufacturer of Silenor, was acquired by Pernix, which hopes to eventually pursue over-the-counter approval.

Bottom Line:
Clinically and pharmacologically, Silenor at 3 mg–6 mg/nightly differs very little from 10 mg/nightly of the generic doxepin, available at a fraction of the price. However, its approval and availability serves as a good reminder that low-dose TCAs may be used as sedatives for their antihistaminic and anticholinergic activity. Silenor/doxepin may be a good agent to put in your arsenal, particularly for those patients in whom you want to avoid benzodiazepines or Z-drugs. There appears to be no good reason to use the much more expensive branded product; stick to the low-dose generic.

ESZOPICLONE (Lunesta) Fact Sheet [G]

FDA Indications:
Insomnia (sleep onset and sleep maintenance).

Off-Label Uses:
None.

Dosage Forms:
Tablets (G): 1 mg, 2 mg, 3 mg.

Dosage Guidance:
Start 1 mg QHS; may ↑ to max 3 mg QHS. Use lower doses in elderly (max 2 mg QHS). Take immediately before falling asleep and with at least 7–8 hours before planned awakening time. Avoid administering with a high-fat meal (delays onset of effect).

Monitoring: No routine monitoring recommended unless clinical picture warrants.

Cost: $

Side Effects:
- Most common: Somnolence, headache, unpleasant taste, dizziness, dry mouth.
- Serious but rare: Anaphylaxis, complex sleep-related behavior (sleep-driving, cooking, eating, phone calls).

Mechanism, Pharmacokinetics, and Drug Interactions:
- Selective GABA-A alpha-1 subunit agonist.
- Metabolized primarily through CYP3A4 and 2E1; t ½: 6 hours (9 hours in elderly).
- Avoid concomitant use with other CNS depressants, including alcohol (additive effects). Potent CYP3A4 inhibitors (eg, fluvoxamine, erythromycin) may increase effects of eszopiclone significantly, whereas CYP3A4 inducers (eg, carbamazepine) may decrease eszopiclone levels; adjust eszopiclone dosing.

Clinical Pearls:
- Schedule IV controlled substance.
- Non-benzodiazepine in structure, but binds to the GABA-benzodiazepine receptor complex like benzodiazepines do; selective for the alpha receptor subtype (causing hypnotic effects but none of the other pharmacologic effects of benzodiazepines); one of the Z-drugs. Eszopiclone is the S-enantiomer of zopiclone (a hypnotic agent available in other countries).
- Unlike benzodiazepines, eszopiclone does not disrupt sleep architecture (stages).
- Taking after a large, high-fat meal will delay its onset of action (by about an hour). Because of its rapid onset of action, eszopiclone should be taken immediately before bedtime or once difficulty falling asleep has occurred.
- Higher doses increase next-day impairment of driving and alertness.

Fun Fact:
Sepracor, the manufacturer, tried to get Lunesta approved in Europe under the brand name Lunivia, but the European agency determined that eszopiclone was too similar to the already-marketed zopiclone to qualify as a patentable product. Sepracor, realizing that it might encounter future generic competition, withdrew its application.

Bottom Line:
Like other Z-drugs, eszopiclone is an effective sedative with less potential for dependence than the benzodiazepines. Dosing is simple and, apart from the bitter aftertaste, its rapid onset and long duration of action make it well accepted among patients. As with all sedatives/hypnotics, nightly use should be discouraged.

FLURAZEPAM (Dalmane) Fact Sheet [G]

FDA Indications:
Insomnia (short term).

Off-Label Uses:
Anxiety disorders; acute mania or psychosis; catatonia.

Dosage Forms:
Capsules (G): 15 mg, 30 mg.

Dosage Guidance:
Start 15 mg QHS. Max 30 mg nightly. Use lower doses in elderly.

Monitoring: No routine monitoring recommended unless clinical picture warrants.

Cost: $

Side Effects:
- Most common: Somnolence, dizziness, weakness, ataxia.
- Serious but rare: Anterograde amnesia, increased fall risk, paradoxical reaction (irritability, agitation), respiratory depression (avoid in patients with sleep apnea).

Mechanism, Pharmacokinetics, and Drug Interactions:
- Binds to benzodiazepine receptors to enhance GABA effects.
- Metabolized primarily through CYP3A4; t ½: 40–100 hours.
- Avoid concomitant use with other CNS depressants, including alcohol and opioids (additive effects). Avoid use with potent 3A4 inhibitors (eg, erythromycin, ketoconazole, fluvoxamine) as they may increase flurazepam levels significantly, whereas CYP3A4 inducers (eg, carbamazepine) may decrease flurazepam levels; adjust flurazepam dosing.

Clinical Pearls:
- Schedule IV controlled substance.
- Flurazepam is less favored than temazepam because of active metabolites, long half-life, potential for accumulation, and next-day grogginess.
- Tolerance to sedative effect may develop within 2–4 weeks of use, and benzodiazepines affect sleep architecture; thus, long-term use is discouraged.

Fun Fact:
Advertising for Dalmane in the 1970s featured a nightgown-clad woman trapped inside a giant eyeball sphere, trying to get out. The tagline: "One less concern for your patient with insomnia."

Bottom Line:
We consider temazepam (and lorazepam), not flurazepam, to be first-line agents for insomnia if a benzodiazepine is appropriate for use (short term, minimal risk of abuse).

RAMELTEON (Rozerem) Fact Sheet

FDA Indications:
Insomnia (sleep onset).

Off-Label Uses:
Jet lag; shift-work sleep disorder.

Dosage Forms:
Tablets: 8 mg.

Dosage Guidance:
Start, target, and maximum dose 8 mg QHS, 30 minutes before bedtime. Avoid administering with high-fat meal (delays therapeutic effect by 45 minutes).

Monitoring: No routine monitoring recommended unless clinical picture warrants.

Cost: $$$$

Side Effects:
- Most common: Headache, somnolence, fatigue, dizziness, nausea.
- Serious but rare: Anaphylaxis, angioedema, complex sleep-related behavior (sleep-driving, cooking, eating, phone calls), increased prolactin, abnormal cortisol or testosterone levels.

Mechanism, Pharmacokinetics, and Drug Interactions:
- Melatonin-1 and melatonin-2 receptor agonist.
- Metabolized primarily through CYP1A2 (major), and to a lesser extent CYP2C9 and 3A4; t ½: 1–2.6 hours.
- Avoid concomitant use with CNS depressants (additive effects). Exercise caution in patients taking potent CYP1A2 inhibitors (eg, fluvoxamine), which could increase ramelteon's effects.

Clinical Pearls:
- Because ramelteon's mechanism of action relates to melatonin receptors and regulation of circadian rhythms, it does not cause patients to "feel" sedated. Often patients say that it doesn't start working for several days—however, clinical trials have shown efficacy from the first night of use. It's good to warn patients about this ahead of time, or they may conclude it's ineffective after 1 night and stop using it.
- No evidence of abuse potential or physical dependence.
- Hormonal alterations occur very rarely and usually with high-dose (16 mg in one study) and longer-term use (6–12 months). If unexplained amenorrhea, galactorrhea, decreased libido, or fertility problems occur, consider evaluating patient's prolactin or testosterone levels.

Fun Fact:
Another melatonin agonist, agomelatine, has been studied as an antidepressant, partly because circadian rhythms are disrupted in depression. It is approved overseas, but the manufacturer scrapped its development in the US.

Bottom Line:
A good alternative to benzodiazepines and Z-drugs for patients at risk for drug abuse or dependence. Compared to other hypnotics, ramelteon poses a lower risk for respiratory depression and hangover effect (morning grogginess). A good agent to have in your bag of tricks, but consider the possibility of rare hormonal effects. Also consider that over-the-counter melatonin (which ramelteon mimics) may do the same job at a lower price.

SUVOREXANT (Belsomra) Fact Sheet

FDA Indications:
Insomnia (sleep onset and sleep maintenance).

Off-Label Uses:
None.

Dosage Forms:
Tablets: 5 mg, 10 mg, 15 mg, 20 mg.

Dosage Guidance:
Start 10 mg QHS, 30 minutes before bedtime and with at least 7 hours remaining before planned awakening time. If tolerated but not effective, may increase to max 20 mg QHS. For more rapid onset, patients should wait at least an hour after a meal before taking it. Avoid administering within an hour of a high-fat meal (delays therapeutic effect by about 1.5 hours).

Monitoring: No routine monitoring recommended unless clinical picture warrants.

Cost: $$$$

Side Effects:
- Most common: Somnolence, headache, abnormal dreams, dry mouth.
- Serious but rare: Impaired alertness and motor coordination, including impaired driving; sleep paralysis (inability to speak or move for up to a few minutes during the sleep-wake transition), hypnagogic/hypnopompic hallucinations (including vivid and disturbing perceptions), and cataplexy-like symptoms (leg weakness for seconds up to a few minutes both in the nighttime and the daytime) reported, especially at higher doses.

Mechanism, Pharmacokinetics, and Drug Interactions:
- "DORA" or dual orexin (OX1 and OX2) receptor antagonist.
- Metabolized primarily through CYP3A4, with minor contribution from 2C19; t ½: 12 hours.
- Caution with CYP3A4 inhibitors and inducers; suvorexant dose adjustment recommended. Caution with alcohol and other CNS depressants.

Clinical Pearls:
- Schedule IV controlled substance. One study found that drug abusers "liked" suvorexant as much as Ambien.
- Suvorexant has a unique mechanism of action. Unlike other hypnotics, it does not act by stimulating GABA or melatonin receptors or by blocking histamine. Instead, suvorexant blocks orexin receptors (orexins are neurotransmitters that promote wakefulness).
- Risk of next-day impairment increases with dose; caution patients taking 20 mg against next-day driving and other activities requiring mental alertness.

Fun Fact:
Merck expected to gain FDA approval for suvorexant in summer 2013. However, the FDA expressed concerns about safety with the 30 mg–40 mg dosing range Merck was proposing and denied approval. It was finally approved in August 2014 at lower doses.

Bottom Line:
Other than a new mechanism of action, there's not much about suvorexant to recommend. There's no reason to expect it to work any better than the other hypnotics already on the market, and it has the same abuse liability. We're concerned that next-day impairment is a potential side effect at the highest approved dose of 20 mg, particularly since sleepless patients may decide on their own to take even higher doses. It's not a first-line hypnotic.

TEMAZEPAM (Restoril) Fact Sheet [G]

FDA Indications:
Insomnia (short term).

Off-Label Uses:
Anxiety disorders; acute mania or psychosis; catatonia.

Dosage Forms:
Capsules (G): 7.5 mg, 15 mg, 22.5 mg, 30 mg.

Dosage Guidance:
Start 15 mg QHS. Max 30 mg nightly. Use lower doses in elderly.

Monitoring: No routine monitoring recommended unless clinical picture warrants.

Cost: 7.5 mg: $; 22.5 mg: $$$

Side Effects:
- Most common: Somnolence, dizziness, weakness, ataxia.
- Serious but rare: Anterograde amnesia, increased fall risk, paradoxical reaction (irritability, agitation), respiratory depression (avoid in patients with sleep apnea).

Mechanism, Pharmacokinetics, and Drug Interactions:
- Binds to benzodiazepine receptors to enhance GABA effects.
- Metabolized primarily through liver but no CYP450 involvement; t ½: 9–18 hours.
- Avoid concomitant use with other CNS depressants, including alcohol and opioids (additive effects). No risk for CYP450 drug interactions.

Clinical Pearls:
- Schedule IV controlled substance.
- Temazepam has long been a favored hypnotic for the elderly because of the lack of active metabolites, its short half-life, and absence of drug interactions.
- If abruptly discontinued, withdrawal symptoms are usually seen on the first day and last for 5–7 days in patients taking this type of short-intermediate half-life benzodiazepine.
- Tolerance to sedative effect may develop within 2–4 weeks of use, and benzodiazepines affect sleep architecture; thus, long-term use is discouraged.

Fun Fact:
The US Air Force uses temazepam as one of the approved "no-go pills" to help aviators and special duty personnel sleep in support of mission readiness; "ground tests" are required prior to authorization being issued to use the medication in an operational situation.

Bottom Line:
We consider temazepam (and lorazepam) to be first-line agents for insomnia if a benzodiazepine is appropriate for use (short term, minimal risk of abuse).

TRIAZOLAM (Halcion) Fact Sheet [G]

FDA Indications:
Insomnia (short term).

Off-Label Uses:
Anxiety disorders; acute mania or psychosis; catatonia.

Dosage Forms:
Tablets (G): 0.125 mg, 0.25 mg.

Dosage Guidance:
Start 0.25 mg QHS; max 0.5 mg QHS. Take immediately before bedtime. Use lower doses in elderly.

Monitoring: No routine monitoring recommended unless clinical picture warrants.

Cost: $

Side Effects:
- Most common: Drowsiness, headache, dizziness, ataxia.
- Serious but rare: Anterograde amnesia, increased fall risk, paradoxical reaction (irritability, agitation); respiratory depression (avoid in patients with sleep apnea).

Mechanism, Pharmacokinetics, and Drug Interactions:
- Binds to benzodiazepine receptors to enhance GABA effects.
- Metabolized primarily through CYP3A4; t ½: 1.5–5.5 hours.
- Avoid concomitant use with other CNS depressants, including alcohol and opioids (additive effects). Avoid use with potent 3A4 inhibitors (eg, erythromycin, ketoconazole, fluvoxamine) as they may increase triazolam levels significantly, whereas CYP3A4 inducers (eg, carbamazepine) may decrease triazolam levels; adjust triazolam dosing.

Clinical Pearls:
- Schedule IV controlled substance.
- Rapid onset of effect; best to take when already in bed.
- Due to its short half-life, triazolam is not effective for patients who suffer from frequent awakenings or early wakening; mostly useful for sleep onset.
- Rebound insomnia and other withdrawal symptoms are more likely and more severe with a short-acting benzodiazepine such as triazolam.
- Tolerance to sedative effect may develop within 2–4 weeks of use, and benzodiazepines affect sleep architecture; thus, long-term use is discouraged.
- May induce more anterograde amnesia than other benzodiazepines; concomitant use of alcohol or use of higher dose (0.5 mg) increases risk.
- Due to studies that suggest the frequency of severe psychiatric disturbances is higher with triazolam compared to other benzodiazepines, the United Kingdom and Brazil have banned it.

Not-So-Fun Fact:
Serial killer Jeffrey Dahmer used triazolam to sedate his victims.

Bottom Line:
There are far better benzodiazepines (lorazepam, temazepam) to use for insomnia in appropriate patients. We cannot recommend using triazolam; some experts have even suggested that it be banned from the US market given the higher likelihood for adverse effects (anterograde amnesia, psychiatric disturbances).

ZALEPLON (Sonata) Fact Sheet [G]

FDA Indications:
Insomnia (short term, sleep onset).

Off-Label Uses:
None.

Dosage Forms:
Capsules (G): 5 mg, 10 mg.

Dosage Guidance:
Start 10 mg QHS, which is the usual dose for most adults. Max 20 mg QHS in those who tolerate but don't benefit from the usual 10 mg dose. Avoid administering with a high-fat meal (delays onset of effect by 2 hours). Use lower doses in elderly.

Monitoring: No routine monitoring recommended unless clinical picture warrants.

Cost: $

Side Effects:
- Most common: Somnolence, dizziness, headache.
- Serious but rare: Anaphylaxis, complex sleep-related behavior (sleep-driving, cooking, eating, phone calls).

Mechanism, Pharmacokinetics, and Drug Interactions:
- Selective GABA-A alpha-1 subunit agonist.
- Metabolized primarily through aldehyde oxidase and also CYP3A4; t ½: 1 hour.
- Avoid concomitant use with other CNS depressants, including alcohol and opioids (additive effects). Potent CYP3A4 inhibitors (eg, fluvoxamine, erythromycin) may increase effects of zaleplon significantly, whereas CYP3A4 inducers (eg, carbamazepine) may decrease zaleplon levels; adjust zaleplon dosing.

Clinical Pearls:
- Schedule IV controlled substance.
- Patients should take it immediately before going to bed or once they are in bed to minimize amnesic episodes.
- Because of zaleplon's very short half-life, it rarely causes next-day impairment.
- Unlike benzodiazepines, zaleplon does not disrupt normal sleep stages.
- Most useful for sleep initiation disorders; does not substantially increase total sleep time or decrease number of awakenings.
- Classified as a Schedule IV drug, but at therapeutic doses, abuse potential is somewhat less than benzodiazepines. However, abuse potential at high doses (2.5–7.5 times recommended dose) is similar to that of benzodiazepines.
- Fewer withdrawal effects than with benzodiazepines, but abrupt discontinuation, particularly from higher doses, can cause withdrawal symptoms (mostly rebound insomnia).

Fun Fact:
The name "Sonata" calls to mind the classical music composition featuring 3 or 4 movements, much like the phases of sleep.

Bottom Line:
Great for inducing sleep, but not great for sleep maintenance throughout the night. Zaleplon is the only sleeping pill that can be taken at 3 am or 4 am without causing functional impairment when the patient gets out of bed at 7 am or 8 am, although patients should always use caution the next day.

ZOLPIDEM (Ambien) Fact Sheet [G]

FDA Indications:

Insomnia (IR: Short term, sleep onset; CR: Sleep onset and maintenance; Intermezzo: Difficulty falling asleep after middle-of-the-night awakening).

Off-Label Uses:

None.

Dosing:

- **Tablets (G):** 5 mg, 10 mg.
- **ER tablets (G):** 6.25 mg, 12.5 mg.
- **SL tablets (Edluar):** 5 mg, 10 mg.
- **SL tablets (Intermezzo, G):** 1.75 mg, 3.5 mg.
- **Oral spray (Zolpimist):** 5 mg/spray.

Dosage Guidance:

- Start 10 mg QHS (5 mg in women). ER: Start 12.5 mg QHS (6.25 mg in women). Take immediately before bed, with at least 7–8 hours remaining before planned awakening time. Dose may be increased to max 10 mg (or 12.5 mg ER) QHS if no daytime grogginess. Higher doses may lead to greater abuse potential. Use lower doses in elderly.
- Lower doses of 1.75 mg (women), 3.5 mg (men) SL QHS can be used with ≥4 hours remaining before wake time.

Monitoring: No routine monitoring recommended unless clinical picture warrants.

Cost: IR, ER: $; Intermezzo, Zolpimist: $$; Edluar: $$$$

Side Effects:

- Most common: Headache, somnolence, dizziness, diarrhea.
- Serious but rare: Complex sleep-related behavior (sleep-driving, cooking, eating, phone calls).

Mechanism, Pharmacokinetics, and Drug Interactions:

- Selective GABA-A alpha-1 subunit agonist.
- Metabolized primarily through CYP3A4; t ½: 2.5–3 hours.
- Avoid concomitant use with other CNS depressants, including alcohol and opioids (additive effects). Potent CYP3A4 inhibitors may increase effects of zolpidem, whereas CYP3A4 inducers (eg, carbamazepine) may decrease zolpidem levels; adjust zolpidem dosing.

Clinical Pearls:

- Schedule IV controlled substance.
- Unlike benzodiazepines, zolpidem does not disrupt normal sleep stages.
- At therapeutic doses, abuse potential is somewhat less than with benzodiazepines.
- Less withdrawal effects than with benzodiazepines, but abrupt discontinuation, particularly from higher doses, can cause withdrawal symptoms (mostly rebound insomnia).
- CR formulation: The dual layer allows some medication to be released immediately, with the rest released gradually, resulting in higher levels through the night.

Fun Fact:

Bioavail Labs received FDA approval for an orally disintegrating tablet form of zolpidem called Tovalt in 2007. It has since been discontinued due to poor sales.

Bottom Line:

Good hypnotic that can also help with sleep maintenance, particularly in the ER formulation. The "new" lower-dose version is simply a patent extender, and we find it difficult to justify the higher cost (use generic zaleplon instead for middle-of-the-night awakening).

Mood Stabilizers

GENERAL PRESCRIBING TIPS

There are many medications that we use to treat bipolar disorder. In this chapter, we focus on meds traditionally known as "mood stabilizers"—agents effective not only for acute episodes of mania or depression, but also for preventing cycling (also known as maintenance treatment of bipolar disorder).

In managing bipolar disorder, manic episodes are usually the most straightforward to treat. In fact, many medications qualify as anti-manic agents: Lithium, valproic acid (VPA), carbamazepine, oxcarbazepine, most atypical antipsychotics, typical antipsychotics (in 1974, chlorpromazine was the second drug approved for acute mania after lithium), and benzodiazepines are all effective, owing to their sedative effect.

Bipolar depression, on the other hand, is more challenging as we have fewer proven strategies. Using antidepressants alone may increase cycling by inducing a "switch" into mania, even though, for better or for worse, it is a strategy often employed. One rigorous study (Systematic Treatment Enhancement Program for Bipolar Disorder, or STEP-BD) found that adding bupropion or paroxetine to a mood stabilizer provided no additional benefit. The medications that have received FDA indications for the treatment of bipolar depression include the combination of fluoxetine and olanzapine (Symbyax), quetiapine (Seroquel), and lurasidone (Latuda). In addition, there are data supporting the use of aripiprazole (Abilify) as well as lithium in bipolar depression.

Maintenance treatment of bipolar disorder should include a mood stabilizer with a proven record of reducing cycling and increasing the time period between acute episodes. Only a few medications have such a record. These include lithium (more effective at preventing mania than depression), lamotrigine (more effective at preventing depression than mania), and some atypical antipsychotics (olanzapine, aripiprazole, quetiapine, and ziprasidone, all more effective at preventing mania than depression). The anticonvulsants VPA and carbamazepine are commonly used as maintenance treatment. Although they are not indicated by the FDA for this purpose, APA treatment guidelines permit VPA and carbamazepine as first-line agents for maintenance treatment of bipolar disorder.

Class Warnings

Several mood stabilizers are also classified as anticonvulsants, and you should note that the FDA issued a black box warning regarding suicide for anticonvulsants as a class. The warning is based on pooled analysis of 199 trials involving various anti-epileptics (regardless of indication) that showed an increased risk of suicidal thoughts/behavior (incidence rate: 0.43% of treated patients compared to 0.24% of patients receiving placebo). The risk was observed as early as 1 week after initiation and continued through duration of trials (most trials ≤24 weeks). The risk was higher for patients with seizure disorders compared to those receiving anticonvulsants for other indications.

Another class warning for the anticonvulsants regards a potentially serious, sometimes fatal multi-organ hypersensitivity reaction syndrome (drug rash with eosinophilia and systemic symptoms, or DRESS), which has been reported with some antiepileptic drugs (rare). Symptoms may include fever, rash, and/or lymphadenopathy; monitor for signs and symptoms of possible disparate manifestations associated with lymphatic, hepatic, renal, and/or hematologic organ systems. Early symptoms of hypersensitivity reaction (eg, lymphadenopathy, fever) may occur without rash. If this occurs, discontinuation and conversion to alternate therapy may be required.

TABLE 11: Mood Stabilizers

Generic Name (Brand Name) Year FDA Approved for Bipolar Disorder or Mania *[G] denotes generic availability*	Relevant FDA Indication(s)	Available Strengths (mg)	Usual Dosage Range (starting–max) (mg)
Carbamazepine (Carbatrol, Epitol, Equetro, Tegretol, Tegretol XR, Teril) [G] 2004	Bipolar disorder (Equetro: Acute mania)	CH: 100, 200 IR: 100, 200, 300, 400 ER: 100, 200, 300, 400 Oral solution: 100 mg/5 mL	200 BID–800 BID
Lamotrigine (Lamictal, Lamictal CD, Lamictal ODT, Lamictal XR) [G] 2003	Bipolar disorder (maintenance)	IR: 5, 25, 50, 100, 150, 200, 250 CH: 2, 5, 25 ODT: 25, 50, 100, 200 ER: 25, 50, 100, 200, 250, 300	25 QD–100 BID 25 QD–50 BID if on VPA
Lithium (Lithobid) [G] 1970	Acute mania Bipolar maintenance	IR: 150, 300, 600 ER: 300, 450 Oral solution: 300 mg/5 mL	300–600 QHS–1200 BID
Oxcarbazepine (Trileptal, Oxtellar XR) [G] 2000	Not approved for any bipolar indication	IR: 150, 300, 600 ER: 150, 300, 600 Oral suspension: 300 mg/5 mL	300 BID–1200 BID
Valproic acid (Depakene, Depakote, Depakote ER, Depakote Sprinkles) [G] 1995	Bipolar disorder (acute mania)	IR: 250 Liquid: 250 mg/5 mL DR: 125, 250, 500 ER: 250, 500	250–500 QHS–2000 BID

CH = chewable, IR = immediate release, ER = extended release, ODT = orally disintegrating tablet, DR = delayed release

CARBAMAZEPINE (Tegretol) Fact Sheet [G]

FDA Indications:
Bipolar disorder (Equetro: Acute mania); seizures; trigeminal neuralgia.

Off-Label Uses:
Bipolar maintenance; impulse control disorders; violence and aggression.

Dosage Forms:
- **Chewable tablets (G):** 100 mg, 200 mg (scored).
- **Tablets (Tegretol, Epitol, G):** 100 mg, 200 mg, 300 mg, 400 mg (scored).
- **ER tablets (Tegretol XR, G):** 100 mg, 200 mg, 400 mg.
- **ER capsules (Equetro, Carbatrol, G):** 100 mg, 200 mg, 300 mg.
- **Oral solution (Tegretol, Teril, G):** 100 mg/5 mL.

Dosage Guidance:
Bipolar disorder: Start at 200 mg BID and gradually ↑ by 200 mg/day every 3–4 days, to target 400 mg–600 mg BID (guided by clinical response). Max 800 mg BID. Dosing is the same for IR and ER versions of carbamazepine; both are BID.

Monitoring: Carbamazepine level, complete blood count, sodium, liver function test, pregnancy test, HLA-B*1502 in Asians.

Cost: IR: $; ER: $$

Side Effects:
- Most common: Dizziness, somnolence, nausea, headache. (ER versions may cause fewer side effects in some patients, but the evidence is not clear.)
- Serious but rare: Hematologic abnormalities including agranulocytosis, aplastic anemia, neutropenia, leukopenia, thrombocytopenia, and pancytopenia reported; hepatic complications including slight increases in hepatic enzymes, cholestatic and hepatocellular jaundice, hepatitis and (rarely) hepatic failure, hyponatremia, SIADH; rash (5%–10%), including exfoliation, reported. Severe reactions including toxic epidermal necrolysis and Stevens-Johnson syndrome are rare, but can be fatal.

Mechanism, Pharmacokinetics, and Drug Interactions:
- Sodium channel blocker.
- Metabolized primarily through CYP3A4; t ½: 15 hours (initially 25–65 hours, but induces its own metabolism within 2–4 weeks and then stabilizes).
- High potential for significant interactions: Potent inducer of CYP1A2, CYP2B6, CYP2C19, CYP2C8, CYP2C9, CYP3A4, P-glycoprotein; use caution with medications significantly metabolized through these pathways as their levels may become subtherapeutic; caution in patients taking strong CYP3A4 inducers or inhibitors that can affect carbamazepine levels.
- Avoid concomitant use with oral contraceptives (can lower serum levels of these contraceptives and cause unplanned pregnancies) and with clozapine (additive risk of agranulocytosis).

Clinical Pearls:
- Therapeutic levels: 4 mcg/mL–12 mcg/mL in seizure disorders. Studies in bipolar haven't shown correlation between levels and clinical response, so it's best dosed clinically.
- Lab monitoring: Baseline and periodic (at 6 weeks and every 3 months) CBC and LFTs.
- Patients of Asian descent should be screened for the variant HLA-B*1502 allele prior to starting carbamazepine; this variant is associated with significantly increased risk of developing Stevens-Johnson syndrome and/or toxic epidermal necrolysis. Avoid use in such patients.

Fun Fact:
Carbamazepine may cause a false-positive serum TCA screen—indeed, its chemical structure contains the familiar tricyclic nucleus common to all TCAs.

Bottom Line:
Equetro is the only FDA-approved formulation for bipolar disorder, but use of other formulations would result in the same effects at a much lower price. However, we do not recommend carbamazepine as a first-line treatment for bipolar disorder due to its side effect profile and high likelihood of significant interactions.

LAMOTRIGINE (Lamictal) Fact Sheet [G]

FDA Indications:
Bipolar disorder (maintenance) in adults; seizures in adults and children.

Off-Label Uses:
Bipolar depression; neuropathic pain; major depression.

Dosage Forms:
- **Tablets (G):** 5 mg, 25 mg, 50 mg, 100 mg, 150 mg, 200 mg, 250 mg (scored).
- **Chewable tablets (Lamictal CD, G):** 2 mg, 5 mg, 25 mg.
- **Orally disintegrating tablets (Lamictal ODT, G):** 25 mg, 50 mg, 100 mg, 200 mg.
- **ER tablets (Lamictal XR, G):** 25 mg, 50 mg, 100 mg, 200 mg, 250 mg, 300 mg.

Dosage Guidance:
- Bipolar disorder: Start 25 mg QD for 2 weeks, ↑ to 50 mg QD for 2 weeks, then 100 mg QD; max 200 mg/day.
- Patients on valproic acid: Start 25 mg QOD (every other day) for 2 weeks, ↑ to 25 mg QD for 2 weeks, then 50 mg QD; max 100 mg/day (VPA doubles lamotrigine levels).
- Dosing is the same with all versions of lamotrigine.

Monitoring: No routine monitoring recommended unless clinical picture warrants.

Cost: IR: $; ER: $$$

Side Effects:
- Most common: Dizziness, headache, nausea, sedation, benign rash (7%).
- Serious but rare: Skin reactions (black box warning): Severe, potentially life-threatening skin rashes requiring hospitalization reported; incidence is higher in pediatric patients; risk increased by co-administration with valproic acid, higher than recommended starting doses, and exceeding recommended dose titration. The majority of cases occur in the first 8 weeks, but isolated cases may occur beyond 8 weeks or even in patients without risk factors. Discontinue at first sign of rash and do not reinitiate unless rash is clearly not drug-related; rare cases of Stevens-Johnson syndrome, toxic epidermal necrolysis, and angioedema reported.

Mechanism, Pharmacokinetics, and Drug Interactions:
- Sodium channel blocker.
- Metabolism primarily hepatic (non-P450); t ½: 25–33 hours (with VPA 48–70 hours; with carbamazepine 13–14 hours).
- Caution with enzyme-inducing medications (eg, carbamazepine), which may decrease lamotrigine levels. Caution with hormonal contraceptives, which may decrease lamotrigine levels; lamotrigine maintenance dose may need to be increased (twofold). Gradual increases of lamotrigine levels may occur during the inactive "pill-free" week. Lamotrigine may decrease levels of some hormonal contraceptives (greater effect with estrogens than progestins); alternative birth control methods should be considered. Valproic acid may double lamotrigine levels, necessitating dosage adjustments (as above).

Clinical Pearls:
- Lamotrigine is useful for the maintenance treatment of bipolar disorder, with best efficacy in the prophylaxis of depressive episodes. Not useful in acute episodes.
- If lamotrigine has been stopped/missed >5 half-lives (see above), consider restarting according to initial dosing recommendations to minimize rash risk.

Fun Fact:
The first FDA-approved drug for bipolar disorder (not just acute mania) since lithium, a drug approved more than 30 years earlier (2003 for lamotrigine; 1970 for lithium).

Bottom Line:
Use lamotrigine for maintenance treatment of bipolar disorder, especially to prevent depressive episodes.

LITHIUM (Lithobid) Fact Sheet [G]

FDA Indications:

Acute mania; bipolar disorder (maintenance) in children and adults.

Off-Label Uses:

Bipolar depression; treatment-resistant depression; neutropenia; vascular headache.

Dosage Forms:

- **Capsules (lithium carbonate, G):** 150 mg, 300 mg, 600 mg.
- **Tablets (lithium carbonate, G):** 300 mg.
- **ER tablets (Lithobid, G):** 300 mg.
- **ER tablets (Eskalith CR, G):** 450 mg (scored).
- **Oral solution (lithium citrate, G):** 300 mg/5 mL.

Dosage Guidance:

Bipolar: Start 300 mg–600 mg QHS; gradually ↑ to target serum lithium level of 0.8 mEq/L (usually 900 mg–1200 mg/day). Can be dosed BID–TID or all QHS. Max 2400 mg/day.

Monitoring: Lithium level, TSH, BUN/creatinine, pregnancy test, ECG if cardiac disease.

Cost: IR, ER: $

Side Effects:

- Most common: Nausea/diarrhea (take with meals, split dosing, switch to ER), fine tremor (lower dose or use propranolol), polyuria/excessive thirst (dose all at bedtime), memory problems, weight gain, hypothyroidism (7%–8%; 9 times more common in women), acne or worsening psoriasis, benign increase in WBC.
- Serious but rare: Chronic use may result in diminished renal concentrating ability (nephrogenic diabetes insipidus); usually reverses when discontinued or treat with hydrochlorothiazide 25 mg–50 mg/day or amiloride 5 mg–10 mg twice daily. Cardiac: Bradycardia, cardiac arrhythmia, flattened or inverted T waves, sinus node dysfunction may occur rarely.

Mechanism, Pharmacokinetics, and Drug Interactions:

- Alters neuronal sodium transport.
- Eliminated by kidneys; t ½: 18–24 hours.
- Drugs that ↑ lithium levels: "**N**o **ACE** in the **H**ole" (**N**SAIDs, **ACE** inhibitors, and **H**CTZ); excess sweating can ↑ levels; low-sodium diet may ↑ lithium levels. Caffeine may ↓ levels.

Clinical Pearls:

- Check lithium level, TSH/T4, BUN/Cr, electrolytes after 1 week of treatment, at 1–2 months, then every 6 to 12 months. Target levels for acute mania: 0.8–1.2 mEq/L; maintenance: 0.6–1.0 mEq/L; toxicity >1.5 mEq/L but may see signs at lower levels, especially in elderly.
- An increase or decrease of 300 mg/day will change serum level by roughly 0.25±0.1 mEq/L.
- Dehydration: Use with caution in patients with significant fluid loss (protracted sweating, diarrhea, or prolonged fever); temporary reduction or discontinuation may be necessary.

Fun Fact:

The soft drink 7-Up was originally called "Bib-Label Lithiated Lemon-Lime Soda" and contained lithium until 1950.

Bottom Line:

Lithium remains the gold standard for bipolar disorder and is likely underutilized today. It is more useful for euphoric mania than for mixed and rapid-cycling types of bipolar disorder, but it is effective for depressive episodes and maintenance treatment of bipolar disorder. It is also known for its anti-suicide effects in bipolar and unipolar mood disorders. Although it is not free from side effects, most common effects can be managed quite well.

OXCARBAZEPINE (Trileptal) Fact Sheet [G]

FDA Indications:
Seizure disorders in adults and children.

Off-Label Uses:
Bipolar disorder.

Dosage Forms:
- **Tablets (G):** 150 mg, 300 mg, 600 mg (scored).
- **Oral suspension (G):** 300 mg/5 mL.
- **ER tablets (Oxtellar XR):** 150 mg, 300 mg, 600 mg.

Dosage Guidance:
Bipolar disorder (off-label): Start 300 mg BID; ↑ by 300 mg/day every 3 days or 600 mg/day weekly to target dose 600–1200 mg BID. Max 2400 mg/day. No data on use of XR for bipolar disorder; caution as higher doses of XR likely needed when converting from IR to XR (not interchangeable on dose-for-dose basis).

Monitoring: Sodium, HLA-B*1502 in Asians.

Cost: IR: $; ER: $$$$

Side Effects:
- Most common: Dizziness; somnolence, headache, ataxia, nausea, vomiting.
- Serious but rare: Potentially serious, sometimes fatal, dermatologic reactions (eg, Stevens-Johnson, toxic epidermal necrolysis) reported; monitor for skin reactions. Rare cases of anaphylaxis and angioedema reported, even after initial dosing; permanently discontinue should symptoms occur.
- Use caution in patients with previous hypersensitivity to carbamazepine (cross-sensitivity occurs in 25%–30%). Clinically significant hyponatremia (serum sodium <125 mmol/L) may develop (1%–3%; higher rate than with carbamazepine); monitor serum sodium, particularly during first 3 months of therapy, especially in patients at risk for hyponatremia.

Mechanism, Pharmacokinetics, and Drug Interactions:
- Sodium channel blocker and neuronal membrane stabilizer.
- Metabolized primarily through CYP450; potent inducer of CYP3A4 and inhibitor of CYP2C19; t ½: 2 hours (9 hours for active metabolite).
- No auto-induction of metabolism and fewer interactions than with carbamazepine. However, there is still potential for interactions. Avoid concomitant use with medications metabolized by CYP3A4 since oxcarbazepine may reduce their levels. Oxcarbazepine may reduce efficacy of oral contraceptives; nonhormonal measures recommended.

Clinical Pearls:
- Oxcarbazepine is the 10-keto analog of carbamazepine (its "chemical cousin"); it is thought of as a kinder, gentler carbamazepine due to its more favorable side effect and drug interaction profile.
- Not bioequivalent to carbamazepine. Increase total daily dose by 20%–30% if switching from carbamazepine to oxcarbazepine.
- Patients of Asian descent should be screened for the variant HLA-B*1502 allele prior to starting oxcarbamazepine; this variant may increase risk of developing Stevens-Johnson syndrome and/or toxic epidermal necrolysis. Avoid use in such patients.

Fun Fact:
While first synthesized in 1965, oxcarbazepine first appeared on the US market in 2000. In 2010, Novartis pleaded guilty to marketing oxcarbazepine for non-FDA approved uses, including neuropathic pain and bipolar disorder, in 2000 and 2001.

Bottom Line:
Compared to carbamazepine, oxcarbazepine poses less concern for drug interactions and hepatic/hematologic toxicities, and does not require serum level monitoring. However, due to the paucity of efficacy data in bipolar disorder, it is reserved for second-line use after lithium and valproic acid.

VALPROIC ACID (Depakote) Fact Sheet [G]

FDA Indications:

Bipolar disorder (acute mania); migraine prophylaxis; seizures.

Off-Label Uses:

Bipolar maintenance; impulse control disorders; violence and aggression.

Dosage Forms:

- **Capsules (valproic acid, G):** 250 mg.
- **Oral liquid (Depakene, G):** 250 mg/5 mL.
- **Tablets (delayed release) (Depakote, G):** 125 mg, 250 mg, 500 mg.
- **Capsules (delayed release) (Depakote Sprinkles, G):** 125 mg.
- **ER tablets (Depakote ER, G):** 250 mg, 500 mg.

Dosage Guidance:

- Acute mania: Start 250 mg–500 mg QHS; ↑ rapidly to effective dose (serum level 50 mcg/mL–125 mcg/mL, target 1000 mg–1500 mg/day); max 4000 mg/day, or 60 mg/kg.
- When converting from regular Depakote to Depakote ER, be aware that patients will get about 20% less valproic acid with the ER formulation.

Monitoring: Valproic acid level, liver function tests, CBC for platelets, pregnancy test, ammonia if confusion.

Cost: DR: $; ER: $$

Side Effects:

- Most common: Somnolence, nausea, fatigue, dizziness, hair loss, tremor, thrombocytopenia (up to 24% of patients; dose-related; reversible).
- Serious but rare: Hepatotoxicity—rare idiosyncratic reaction, not dose-related; most cases occur within 3 months; risk factors: age <2 years, multiple anticonvulsants, and presence of neurologic disease in addition to epilepsy. Asymptomatic elevations of liver enzymes may occur, not necessarily associated with hepatic dysfunction. Pancreatitis (rare but potentially fatal). Polycystic ovary syndrome (PCOS) in about 10% of women. Hyperammonemia, encephalopathy (sometimes fatal) reported and may present with normal liver enzymes.

Mechanism, Pharmacokinetics, and Drug Interactions:

- Sodium channel blocker.
- Metabolized primarily by liver with only minimal (10%) role of CYP450 enzymes (2A6, 2B6, 2C9); t ½: 9–16 hours.
- VPA causes ↑ levels of lamotrigine and risk for rash. Taking with topiramate can lead to encephalopathy.

Clinical Pearls:

- ER tablets have 10%–20% less fluctuation in serum concentration than delayed release tablets. Divalproex sodium ER and DR tablets are *not* bioequivalent; increase total daily dose by 10%–20% if switching from DR to ER.
- Elevations of ammonia can often occur at normal doses and serum levels of VPA. Reducing dose when clinically appropriate typically reverses ammonia elevation. Treating with L-carnitine is also effective.
- Once steady state levels reached (within 2–4 days of initiation or dose adjustment), trough serum levels should be drawn just before the next dose (ER/DR preparations) or before the morning dose (for immediate release preparations).

Fun Fact:

Valproic acid was first synthesized in 1882 by B.S. Burton as an analogue of valeric acid, found naturally in valerian.

Bottom Line:

VPA is the go-to antimanic agent for acute manic episodes, featuring faster onset of response and better adverse effect profile compared to lithium, fewer drug interactions than carbamazepine, and efficacy for rapid cycling and relapse prevention.

Natural Treatments

GENERAL PRESCRIBING TIPS

If you're interested in natural treatments (also known as complementary and alternative medicine, or CAM), you will likely recommend various strategies other than the 8 medications we cover in this section. These would include exercise (helpful for depression and for preventing cognitive impairment), light therapy (for seasonal affective disorder), massage, meditation, and other modalities.

We have included fact sheets on those natural products that have been shown to be effective via standard randomized controlled trials. Some natural products not included here might be effective but have not been adequately tested vs placebo.

Because most of these products are not regulated by the FDA, there are quality control issues. The amount of active constituents can vary not only from brand to brand, but also from batch to batch, and some products may be adulterated with other herbs, chemicals, drugs, or toxins. We recommend that patients stick to well-known brands sold by trusted retailers.

For additional information, you may also find these resources helpful:

- NIH National Center for Complementary and Integrative Health: https://nccih.nih.gov/health/herbsataglance.htm
- National Library of Medicine: medlineplus.gov/druginfo/herb_All.html
- Natural Medicines Comprehensive Database (requires subscription): http://naturaldatabase.therapeuticresearch.com
- ConsumerLab (requires subscription): http://www.consumerlab.com/

TABLE 12: Natural Treatments

Name (Brand Name, if applicable)	Commonly Available Strengths (mg)	Reported Uses in Psychiatry	Usual Dosage Range (starting–max) (mg)
L-methylfolate (Deplin and others)	0.4, 0.8, 1, 3, 5, 7.5, 15	Depression (adjunct)	15
L-tryptophan	500	Depression	300–2000
Melatonin	0.5, 1, 2.5, 3, 5, 10	Insomnia	1–20
N-acetylcysteine	500, 600, 750, 1000	OCD, trichotillomania, nail biting, skin picking	1200–2400
Omega-3 fatty acids (fish oil)	500, 1000, 1200	Depression (unipolar, bipolar)	500–2000
S-adenosyl-L-methionine (SAMe)	100, 200, 400	Depression	800 BID
St. John's wort	100, 300, 450	Depression	300 TID
Vitamin D	1000 IU, 2000 IU, 5000 IU, 10,000 IU (as D3)	Depression	1000–5000 IU

L-METHYLFOLATE (Deplin) Fact Sheet

FDA Indications:

None.

Off-Label Uses:

Adjunctive treatment for depression (considered a "medical food product" by the FDA, not an FDA-approved drug product, although available as prescription only).

Dosage Forms:

- **Capsules (Deplin):** 7.5 mg, 15 mg.
- **Tablets and capsules (various other L-methylfolate products):** 0.4 mg, 0.8 mg, 1 mg, 3 mg, 5 mg.

Dosage Guidance:

Depression (Deplin only): Start 7.5 mg QD; target and max dose 15 mg/day.

Monitoring: No routine monitoring recommended unless clinical picture warrants.

Cost: G: $$; Deplin: $$$

Side Effects:

- Most common: Not well known; likely well tolerated.
- Serious but rare: Folic acid supplementation may mask symptoms of vitamin B12 deficiency (administration of folic acid may reverse the hematological signs of B12 deficiency, including megaloblastic anemia, while not addressing neurological manifestations). L-methylfolate may be less likely than folic acid to mask B12 deficiency, though the possibility should be considered.

Mechanism, Pharmacokinetics, and Drug Interactions:

- May enhance synthesis of monoamine neurotransmitters.
- No typical drug metabolism pathway as it is naturally stored and used by body; t ½: 3 hours.
- Drug interactions generally unlikely, although L-methylfolate may decrease anticonvulsant levels (including carbamazepine and valproic acid). Drugs that lower folate, such as anticonvulsants (including carbamazepine, valproic acid, and lamotrigine), may necessitate higher doses of L-methylfolate.

Clinical Pearls:

- Dietary folic acid is normally transformed to L-methylfolate by the enzyme MTHFR, and L-methylfolate is necessary for the synthesis of monoamines (serotonin, norepinephrine, dopamine). The marketing pitch for prescribing Deplin is that in about 50% of the population, genetic variations impair the function of MTHFR, leading to low levels of methylfolate. A recent review of the data on one of these genetic polymorphisms (called C677T) found that overall, it did not put people at any higher risk of depression (in fact, schizophrenia was more common).
- A few small studies over the years have shown that both folate (over the counter) and L-methylfolate may be somewhat helpful as adjunctive agents in the treatment of depression, particularly in those with low baseline folate levels.

Fun Fact:

"Medical foods" are foods that are specially formulated and intended for the dietary management of a disease with distinctive nutritional needs that cannot be met by normal diet alone. These include total parenteral nutrition as well as nasogastric tube feeds and oral rehydration products. Depression has no accepted distinctive nutritional needs.

Bottom Line:

Though the data are not robust, folate supplementation *might* be effective for some patients with depression, but we recommend that patients try the cheap stuff (folic acid) before springing for Deplin (L-methylfolate).

L-TRYPTOPHAN Fact Sheet

FDA Indications:
None.

Off-Label Uses:
Depression; premenstrual dysphoric disorder (PMDD); smoking cessation.

Dosage Forms:
Capsules: 500 mg.

Dosage Guidance:
For depression, 300 mg/day in combination with antidepressants has been used. For other uses, dose is typically 500 mg–1000 mg BID or 500 mg TID. PMDD dosing studied is 6 g/day.

Monitoring: No routine monitoring recommended unless clinical picture warrants.

Cost: $$

Side Effects:
- Most common: Abdominal pain, nausea, vomiting, diarrhea, flatulence, headache.
- Serious but rare: Over 1,500 reports of eosinophilia-myalgia syndrome (EMS) and 37 deaths were reported in the US, leading to it being pulled from the market in 1990; nearly all cases were tied to contaminated batches out of Japan. Symptoms of EMS include eosinophilia, fatigue, myalgia, neuropathy, rash, and inflammation. There have been no reported recurrences of these reactions since that outbreak.

Mechanism, Pharmacokinetics, and Drug Interactions:
- Essential amino acid found in plant and animal proteins. Absorbed from dietary protein sources and converted to 5-hydroxytryptophan (5-HTP) and then to serotonin (5-hydroxytryptamine).
- Metabolized by non P450 liver pathway; t ½: 3–4 hours.
- Combining with serotonergic antidepressants may increase risk of serotonin syndrome. Avoid use with MAOIs.

Clinical Pearls:
- Best efficacy in PMDD and smoking cessation. Evidence for use in depression is limited but suggestive.
- L-tryptophan has also been studied in attention deficit hyperactivity disorder, anxiety, depression, fibromyalgia, insomnia, and migraines, but there is insufficient evidence to support these uses.
- While both can cross the blood-brain barrier, L-tryptophan more readily does so than 5-HTP.
- Combination formulations are sold as "serotonin boosters" and include amino acids (tryptophan, 5-HTP, SAMe), vitamins (B6, B9, B12, C, D), minerals (magnesium, zinc) and herbs (theanine, curcumin, garcinia, rhodiola). These formulations all have extremely limited evidence to support efficacy in depression.

Fun Fact:
Especially around Thanksgiving, many will talk about "turkey coma" as a result of ingesting too much tryptophan contained in turkey. Actually, the drowsiness is more likely due to all the carbs eaten with the turkey. Turkey has no more tryptophan than other meats.

Bottom Line:
The evidence base to support using L-tryptophan in depression is extremely limited, but more and more patients are turning to it, especially in combination "serotonin boost" products being marketed today. We recommend sticking to the serotonergic agents we know to be safe and effective: SSRIs and SNRIs.

MELATONIN Fact Sheet

FDA Indications:

None.

Off-Label Uses:

Insomnia; jet lag; work-shift sleep disorder.

Dosage Forms:

Supplied over the counter (OTC) in various forms including liquid, tablets, capsules, sublingual, and time-release formulations; usually in 0.5 mg, 1 mg, 2.5 mg, 3 mg, 5 mg, and 10 mg.

Dosage Guidance:

- Insomnia (adults): 0.5 mg–20 mg in early evening. Emerging data suggest lower doses are effective; start low (0.5 mg–1 mg) and gradually increase to desired effect ("normal" melatonin levels vary widely among individuals, and the same dose can induce different levels depending on age or health).
- For jet lag, 1 mg–3 mg on day of departure at a time that corresponds to the anticipated bedtime at arrival destination, followed by 1 mg–3 mg at bedtime for next 3–5 days.

Monitoring: No routine monitoring recommended unless clinical picture warrants.

Cost: $

Side Effects:

- Most common: Generally well tolerated in the short term. Drowsiness, headaches, and dizziness most common but at similar rates to placebo; next-day grogginess or irritability (higher doses); vivid dreams or nightmares (higher doses).
- Serious but rare: No serious side effects reported; however, long-term human studies have not been conducted. Theoretically, melatonin may alter other hormones (inhibiting ovulation in women and gonadal development in children and adolescents); avoid use in women who are pregnant or are attempting to become pregnant, and use caution in children.

Mechanism, Pharmacokinetics, and Drug Interactions:

- Melatonin receptor agonist.
- Metabolized primarily through CYP1A2, may inhibit CYP1A2; t ½: 35–50 minutes.
- Some suggest melatonin may reduce glucose tolerance and insulin sensitivity and may ↑ efficacy of calcium channel blockers for blood pressure.

Clinical Pearls:

- Melatonin is secreted from the pineal gland in a 24-hour circadian rhythm. It rises at sunset and peaks in the middle of the night, regulating the normal sleep/wake cycle.
- Melatonin should only be taken in its synthetic form; the "natural" form comes from ground-up cow pineal glands and may spread disease (eg, mad cow disease).
- Melatonin taken at bedtime doesn't seem to affect nocturnal sleep. Taken in the early evening, it appears to be similar to temazepam in hypnotic effect.
- Although melatonin products have been available over the counter in the US since the mid-1990s, many countries require a prescription, and some do not permit its sale.

Fun Fact:

Foods containing melatonin include cherries, bananas, grapes, rice, cereals, herbs, olive oil, wine, and beer.

Bottom Line:

Short-term melatonin treatment appears to only modestly reduce the time it takes to fall asleep (about 12 minutes, which might not be considered clinically relevant) and does not appear to significantly improve overall sleep time. However, some patients report minor improvement in subjective feelings of sleep quality. It may be something to consider using in the short term, particularly in older patients (whose endogenous melatonin levels are lower). It is cheaper than ramelteon (Rozerem); however, like ramelteon, it lacks good long-term safety data, especially with regard to effects on hormones.

N-ACETYLCYSTEINE (NAC) Fact Sheet

FDA Indications:
None.

Off-Label Uses:
Obsessive compulsive disorder (OCD); trichotillomania; nail biting; skin picking.

Dosage Forms:
Capsules: 500 mg, 600 mg, 750 mg, 1000 mg.

Dosage Guidance:
NAC doses studied have ranged from 600 mg to 6000 mg/day, with the majority of the studies using 1200–2400 mg/day. Divide dose BID to minimize GI side effects.

Monitoring: No routine monitoring recommended unless clinical picture warrants.

Cost: $

Side Effects:
- Most common: Usually well tolerated with nausea/vomiting, diarrhea, cramping, flatulence being most common.
- Serious but rare: May exacerbate asthma.

Mechanism, Pharmacokinetics, and Drug Interactions:
- NAC is derived from the amino acid cysteine, a precursor of a key brain antioxidant, glutathione. It works as a glutamate modulator, which may have effects on oxidative stress, mitochondrial dysfunction, inflammatory mediators, neurotransmission, and neural plasticity.
- Metabolized extensively by liver with minimal P450 involvement; t ½: 6 hours.
- No known drug interactions; not likely an issue for the majority of patients.

Clinical Pearls:
- Amino acid derivate with antioxidant properties.
- NAC is most recognized for its use as a treatment for acetaminophen overdose.
- Although NAC has been studied in autism, Alzheimer's, cocaine and cannabis addiction, bipolar disorder, depression, trichotillomania, nail biting, skin picking, obsessive-compulsive disorder (OCD), and schizophrenia, the results are generally mixed. Best data are in patients with OCD, trichotillomania, nail biting, and skin picking (including Prader-Willi syndrome).
- Most patients develop tolerance to GI symptoms, and they go away after a few weeks.
- No long-term data; most studies were 8 weeks long, and a few followed patients for up to 3–6 months.

Fun Fact:
Many of the published studies have come from an individual Australian researcher who holds a patent on a particular formulation of NAC, raising the issue of bias or a potential conflict of interest.

Bottom Line:
The efficacy of NAC in a large number of psychiatric disorders has been investigated. For now, it is best reserved as an add-on for patients only partially responding to SSRIs in treatment for OCD or the other repetitive behaviors involving hair, nails, and skin.

OMEGA-3 FATTY ACIDS (Fish Oil) Fact Sheet

FDA Indications:

High triglycerides (as Lovaza).

Off-Label Uses:

Unipolar and bipolar depression.

Dosage Forms:

- Supplied over the counter in various dosages and formulations; 500 mg, 1000 mg, and 1200 mg softgel capsules most common.
- By prescription only: Lovaza: 1000 mg softgel capsules (GSK). Dosage on label usually reflects fish oil dosage, which is not the same as omega-3 fatty acid dosage (eg, 1000 mg fish oil in some brands may provide 300 mg of omega-3 fatty acids, including EPA and DHA). Dosing recommendations are based on mg of fish oil.

Dosage Guidance:

Effective dose unclear, but studies have used 300 mg to 6 g QD. For depression, start 500 mg/day, increase as tolerated (target dose 1 g–2 g/day); doses >3 g/day should be used cautiously. Dividing dose BID–TID helps with side effect tolerability.

Monitoring: No routine monitoring recommended unless clinical picture warrants.

Cost: $

Side Effects:

- Most common: Well tolerated up to 4 g/day. Nausea, loose stools, fishy aftertaste.
- Serious but rare: Caution in those who are allergic to seafood. Increased risk of bleeding, particularly at higher doses.

Mechanism, Pharmacokinetics, and Drug Interactions:

- Exact mechanism unknown, but may improve cell membrane fluidity and membrane function, change neurotransmitter binding, and promote anti-inflammatory effects.
- Metabolism is hepatic, primarily through CYP450; t ½: Unknown.
- For most patients, drug interactions not likely an issue; however, may prolong bleeding time. Fish oils may lower blood pressure and have additive effects when used with antihypertensives.

Clinical Pearls:

- Fish oils contain eicosapentaenoic acid (EPA) and docosahexaenoic acid (DHA); both are omega-3 fatty acids (which form the lipid bilayers of cell membranes). Although the body can synthesize these fats from alpha-linolenic acid (ALA), this is believed to be inefficient in many people.
- EPA and DHA are derived from fish; ALA is derived from flax seed and other vegetable matter. Mercury accumulates in fish meat more than in fish oil, which might explain the lack of detectable mercury in most fish oil supplements. Also, the manufacturing process that is used to deodorize fish oil supplements seems to lower the levels of PCBs and other contaminants.
- Omega-3 fatty acids have been tested in the treatment of schizophrenia, bipolar disorder, depression, anxiety, obsessive-compulsive disorder, attention deficit hyperactivity disorder, autism, aggression, borderline personality disorder, substance use disorder, anorexia nervosa, and dementia. With the exception of depressive disorders, overall consensus is still lacking for the majority of these uses due to limited sample sizes, selection of patients, doses and formulations used, and duration of study.
- Omega-3 fatty acids appear helpful as augmentation in unipolar depression in some individual studies, but several meta-analyses have not been able to show robust benefit. In positive studies, most benefit seen at 1 g/day with EPA more effective than DHA and more severely ill patients showing greater improvement.

Fun Fact:

Inuit people have been reported to ingest up to 16 g/day (via fish) with no dangerous side effects.

Bottom Line:

The evidence on efficacy in depression is still somewhat conflicting, and the ideal dose has not been clearly established. However, since omega-3 fatty acids are fairly benign and may offer other health benefits, you may consider using them from time to time. Based on the limited data available, the best use of omega-3 fatty acids (particularly 1 g–2 g with at least 60% EPA), in our opinion, is as an adjunct in the treatment of unipolar and bipolar depression. There is not enough evidence to recommend omega-3 fatty acids in other disorders at this time.

S-ADENOSYL-L-METHIONINE (SAMe) Fact Sheet

FDA Indications:
None.

Off-Label Uses:
Depression; osteoarthritis; cirrhosis and fatty liver disease.

Dosage Forms:
Supplied over the counter most often as 100 mg, 200 mg, 400 mg tablets, usually enteric coated.

Dosage Guidance:
Effective dose is variable, but most antidepressant studies have used doses of about 400 mg–1600 mg/day (1600 mg most common), usually divided BID.

Monitoring: No routine monitoring recommended unless clinical picture warrants.

Cost: $

Side Effects:
- Most common: Well tolerated. Higher doses may result in flatulence, nausea, vomiting, diarrhea, constipation, dry mouth, headache, mild insomnia, anorexia, sweating, dizziness, and nervousness. Anxiety and tiredness have occurred in people with depression, and hypomania has occurred in people with bipolar disorder.
- Serious but rare: Theoretical concern of elevated homocysteine since SAMe is converted to this during normal metabolism. No reports to date, but some recommend taking folate and vitamin B supplements anyway.

Mechanism, Pharmacokinetics, and Drug Interactions:
- Methyl group donor that may increase synthesis of neurotransmitters, increase responsiveness of neurotransmitter receptors, and increase fluidity of cell membranes through the production of phospholipids.
- Metabolism similar to endogenous SAMe (transmethylation, trans-sulphuration, and aminopropylation); t ½: 100 minutes.
- No drug interactions reported. Theoretically, serotonin syndrome possible but risk likely minimal.

Clinical Pearls:
- SAMe is produced by our bodies as a derivative of the amino acid methionine. It functions as a methyl donor and is necessary for the production of serotonin and norepinephrine (and in more than 100 other biochemical reactions) throughout virtually all body tissues and fluids. Concentrations are highest in childhood and decrease with age.
- SAMe is difficult to formulate as a stable oral salt, and the FDA halted trials of an investigational prescription product in 1993 due to concerns about tablet dissolution; concerns have been raised that some supplements may also have these problems.

Fun Facts:
SAMe has been available as a dietary supplement in the US since 1999, but it has been used as a prescription drug in Italy since 1979, in Spain since 1985, and in Germany since 1989. Patients in trials of SAMe for depression noted improvement in their arthritis symptoms, suggesting another possible use.

Bottom Line:
Several clinical studies (lasting up to 42 days) have shown that taking SAMe is more effective than placebo and appears to be as effective as TCAs. However, some of these studies are limited by small numbers of patients, inconsistent diagnostic criteria, and short treatment periods. Also, some studies used injectable SAMe rather than oral, so generalizability of findings is a concern. SAMe may have a role as an adjunctive agent in patients who do not respond to antidepressants. Consider using it for those patients with mild to moderate depression who are interested in using alternative therapies, or as an augmentation strategy in partial responders.

ST. JOHN'S WORT Fact Sheet

FDA Indications:
None.

Off-Label Uses:
Depression.

Dosage Forms:
Supplied over the counter most commonly as 100 mg, 300 mg, 450 mg tablets and capsules.

Dosage Guidance:
For mild to moderate depression, most clinical trials have used St. John's wort extract containing 0.3% hypericin and/or 3% hyperforin; most common dose is 300 mg TID. Doses of 1200 mg QD have also been used. Some studies have also used a 0.2% hypericin extract dosed at 250 mg BID. A St. John's wort extract standardized to 5% hyperforin and dosed at 300 mg TID has also been used.

Monitoring: No routine monitoring recommended unless clinical picture warrants.

Cost: $

Side Effects:
- Most common: Well tolerated at recommended doses. Insomnia (decrease dose or take in morning), vivid dreams, restlessness, anxiety, agitation, irritability, gastrointestinal discomfort, diarrhea, fatigue, dry mouth, dizziness, and headache reported. Sexual dysfunction may occur, but less often than with SSRIs.
- Serious but rare: Risk of severe phototoxic skin reactions and photosensitivity at high doses (2–4 grams/day).

Mechanism, Pharmacokinetics, and Drug Interactions:
- Thought to exert antidepressant effects by modulating effects of monoamines, and may inhibit reuptake of these neurotransmitters.
- Metabolized primarily through the liver; t ½: 24–48 hours.
- Avoid concomitant use with serotonergic agents: Rare cases of serotonin syndrome reported. Potent inducer of many CYP450 enzymes (3A4, 2C9, 1A2) and p-glycoprotein transporter, which results in increased metabolism and reduced plasma concentrations of a large number of drugs. St. John's wort can decrease oral contraceptive levels by 13%–15%, resulting in bleeding or unplanned pregnancy; women should use an additional or nonhormonal form of birth control.

Clinical Pearls:
- Also known as *Hypericum perforatum*; active constituents (predominantly hypericin and hyperforin) are derived from the flowering buds.
- St. John's wort is more effective than placebo, likely as effective as low-dose TCAs and SSRIs in milder forms of depression; however, a study in *JAMA* found it no more effective than placebo or sertraline for moderate to severe depression.
- Avoid abrupt discontinuation due to the risk of withdrawal effects.

Fun Facts:
Although not indigenous to Australia and long considered a weed, St. John's wort is now grown as a cash crop, and Australia produces 20% of the world's supply. The use of St. John's wort dates back to the ancient Greeks; Hippocrates documented the medical use of St. John's wort flowers. St. John's wort is so named because it blooms near June 24th, which is the birthday of John the Baptist. "Wort" is an old English word for plant.

Bottom Line:
St. John's wort can be considered an option along with conventional antidepressants for short-term treatment of mild depression; however, be wary of its many drug interactions.

VITAMIN D Fact Sheet

FDA Indications:
None.

Off-Label Uses:
Depression.

Dosage Forms:
Supplied over the counter as vitamin D2 and D3, as tablets, capsules, and softgels in "international units" (IU) dosing. We recommend D3: 1000 IU, 2000 IU, 5000 IU, 10,000 IU.

Dosage Guidance:
Dosing guidelines vary. For depression, use 1000–5000 IU per day.

Monitoring: Periodic vitamin D [25(OH)D] levels.

Cost: $

Side Effects:
- Most common: Well tolerated.
- Serious but rare: Vitamin D toxicity possible but very rare.

Mechanism, Pharmacokinetics, and Drug Interactions:
- Thought to play a role in brain plasticity, neuroimmunomodulation, and inflammation.
- Metabolized by liver and kidneys; t ½: 12–50 days (varies based on level, source, dose, obesity, and race).
- No known significant interactions.

Clinical Pearls:
- Sources of vitamin D include exposure to sunlight, dietary intake, and supplements.
- It's difficult to obtain sufficient daily needs from dietary intake alone. Two types of vitamin D are obtained from dietary sources: D2 (ergocalciferol) from plant sources such as mushrooms and soy milk and D3 (cholecalciferol) from animal sources such as raw fish, mackerel, smoked salmon). D3 is approximately three times stronger than D2.
- Majority of vitamin D is produced through conversion of 7-dehydrocholesterol via ultraviolet B, after penetration of sunlight on the skin, to vitamin D3.
- Vitamin D is metabolized in the liver to 25-hydroxyvitamin D or 25(OH)D and then in the kidneys to its active form calcitriol, or 1,25-dihydroxyvitamin D. Labs will usually report 25(OH)D level with 30–60 ng/mL as normal range, 21–29 ng/mL as insufficiency, and <20 ng/mL as deficiency.
- Several meta-analyses have found no beneficial effects of vitamin D supplementation on depression. When studies were limited to depressed patients with both vitamin D insufficiency at baseline and adequate dosing of supplementation (>800 mg/day), statistically significant benefits were seen.
- Studies in anxiety, psychosis, and dementia have not shown positive results of supplementation.

Fun Fact:
A number of things affect your vitamin D status, including how far away you live from the Equator, the air quality in your community, your skin color, and your use of sunscreen.

Bottom Line:
Vitamin D supplementation may possibly be beneficial in depression, but reserve its use for those who have insufficiency, and have patients take 1000–5000 IU daily.

Novel Anticonvulsants

GENERAL PRESCRIBING TIPS

There's a great tradition in psychiatry of adopting anti-epileptic drugs for use in psychiatric syndromes. In some cases, such as Depakote, Tegretol, and Lamictal, this strategy has yielded effective treatments. But for the 3 drugs covered in this chapter (gabapentin, pregabalin, and topiramate), the payoff has been fairly scant. All 3 were initially touted as having efficacy in bipolar disorder, based on uncontrolled trials. However, subsequent data from randomized controlled trials did not support this indication.

Nonetheless, these drugs have found their places in other spheres, especially disorders related to anxiety. For example, pregabalin is approved for generalized anxiety disorder in parts of Europe. It also has pretty convincing data for effectiveness in helping patients discontinue benzodiazepines. Topiramate seems to have a niche for patients with alcohol dependence and for any patient who wants to lose weight. Gabapentin is a non-addictive alternative to benzodiazepines for anxiety and alcohol dependence.

Oxcarbazepine is covered in our Mood Stabilizers chapter because it has pretty good evidence for the treatment of bipolar disorder. Sharp-eyed readers may recall that we included a fact sheet for tiagabine (Gabitril) in the previous edition of the *Medication Fact Book*. We decided to omit it this time because the data supporting its use in mood or anxiety disorders are very weak, and the drug is associated with side effects including seizures and syncope. If more impressive tiagabine data emerge, it may merit a reappearance in our 5th edition.

Side Effects

The newer anticonvulsants are appealing because they are generally less toxic than the older agents, do not require serum level monitoring, and in most cases have a lower risk of drug interactions.

However, the anti-epileptics have a class warning for increased risk of suicidal thoughts and behavior; this warning stems from pooled analysis of trials (for seizure disorders as well as other indications) that showed a nearly doubled incidence of suicidal thought and behavior (0.43% for anticonvulsants vs 0.24% for placebo).

TABLE 13: Novel Anticonvulsants

Generic Name (Brand Name) Year FDA Approved *[G] denotes generic availability*	Off-Label Psychiatric Uses	Available Strengths (mg)	Usual Dosage Range (starting–max) (mg)
Gabapentin (Neurontin) [G] 1993	Anxiety disorders Withdrawal from alcohol or benzodiazepines Alcohol dependence	Capsule: 100, 300, 400 Tablet: 600, 800 Oral solution: 50 mg/mL ER tablet: 300, 600	100 QHS–300 TID
Pregabalin (Lyrica) 2004	Generalized anxiety disorder Withdrawal from alcohol or benzodiazepines Alcohol dependence	Capsule: 25, 50, 75, 100, 150, 200, 225, 300	75 BID–300 BID
Topiramate (Topamax) [G] 1996	Alcohol dependence Bipolar disorder PTSD Binge-eating disorder Obesity	Tablet: 25, 50, 100, 200 Capsule: 15, 25 ER capsule: 25, 50, 100, 150, 200	25 BID–150 BID

GABAPENTIN (Neurontin) Fact Sheet [G]

FDA Indications:
Partial seizures (Neurontin); post-herpetic neuralgia (Gralise, Neurontin); restless leg syndrome (Horizant).

Off-Label Uses:
Anxiety disorders; withdrawal from alcohol or benzodiazepines; alcohol dependence.

Dosage Forms:
- **Capsules (G):** 100 mg, 300 mg, 400 mg.
- **Tablets (G):** 600 mg, 800 mg.
- **Oral solution (G):** 50 mg/mL.
- **Tablets, ER (Gralise):** 300 mg, 600 mg.
- **Tablets, ER (Horizant):** 300 mg, 600 mg (gabapentin enacarbil, a prodrug with better bioavailability).

Dosage Guidance:
For anxiety (off-label use), start 100 mg QHS and increase as tolerated to 300 mg TID. Max 3600 mg/day (highest doses often used for pain indications). Use lower doses in patients with renal impairment.

Monitoring: No routine monitoring recommended unless clinical picture warrants.

Cost: IR: $; ER: $$$$$

Side Effects:
- Most common: Dizziness, somnolence, ataxia, weight gain.
- Serious but rare: Potentially serious, sometimes fatal multiorgan hypersensitivity (also known as drug reaction with eosinophilia and systemic symptoms, or DRESS).

Mechanism, Pharmacokinetics, and Drug Interactions:
- Blocks voltage-dependent calcium channels and modulates excitatory neurotransmitter release.
- Not metabolized; excreted unchanged by kidneys; t ½: 5–7 hours.
- Few significant drug interactions, although you may see additive sedative effects with other sedating drugs. Analgesic control may be affected when gabapentin is added to opiates, including decreased levels of hydrocodone (Vicodin) or increased levels of morphine.

Clinical Pearls:
- Gabapentin is structurally related to GABA. However, it does not bind to GABA-A or GABA-B receptors, and it does not appear to influence synthesis or uptake of GABA.
- Controlled trials have shown no effect as monotherapy or adjunctive therapy for bipolar disorder.
- Data with acute alcohol or benzodiazepine withdrawal (both inpatient and outpatient) are limited but promising.
- There have been reports of recreational use of gabapentin in correctional facilities, some of which have restricted its use.
- Recreational use and abuse in the general population is also increasing and seems to occur more often with pregabalin than gabapentin, often at supratherapeutic dosing for the euphoric effects. Those with opioid use disorders have much higher gabapentin and pregabalin abuse rates.

Fun Fact:
Gabapentin recently was reclassified as a controlled substance in Kentucky (Schedule V). Prescribers must have a DEA license, and prescriptions will be logged in the state's PDMP database. More states and the federal government likely will follow.

Bottom Line:
Clinicians tend to use gabapentin when they want a non-addictive medication for anxiety and for alcohol dependence. The data for these uses is lukewarm, but not negative. It almost certainly does not work for bipolar disorder per se, though it might help with associated symptoms like anxiety and insomnia. If you have a patient with anxiety plus one of the approved uses (such as neuropathic pain and restless leg syndrome), then it's a particularly good choice.

PREGABALIN (Lyrica) Fact Sheet

FDA Indications:

Diabetic peripheral neuropathy; spinal cord injury–associated neuropathic pain; post-herpetic neuralgia; partial seizures; fibromyalgia.

Off-Label Uses:

Generalized anxiety disorder; withdrawal from alcohol or benzodiazepines; alcohol dependence.

Dosage Forms:

Capsules: 25 mg, 50 mg, 75 mg, 100 mg, 150 mg, 200 mg, 225 mg, 300 mg.

Dosage Guidance:

Start 75 mg BID and ↑ as tolerated to max 300 mg BID (based on trials for generalized anxiety disorder, an off-label use). Use lower doses in renal impairment.

Monitoring: No routine monitoring recommended unless clinical picture warrants.

Cost: $$$$

Side Effects:

- Most common: Peripheral edema, dizziness, somnolence, ataxia, weight gain.
- Serious but rare: Hypersensitivity reactions, including skin redness, blistering, hives, rash, dyspnea, and wheezing. Angioedema, possibly life-threatening, reported; use with caution in patients with a history of angioedema or patients on ACE inhibitors. Increases in CPK and rare cases of rhabdomyolysis reported.

Mechanism, Pharmacokinetics, and Drug Interactions:

- Binds alpha-2 delta subunit of calcium channels and reduces neurotransmitter release.
- Negligible metabolism; mostly excreted unchanged by kidneys; t ½: 6 hours.
- No significant drug interactions, although you may see additive sedative effects with other sedating drugs.

Clinical Pearls:

- Schedule V controlled substance (same category as cough suppressants containing codeine). Following abrupt withdrawal, patients may experience insomnia, nausea, headache, or diarrhea; this may be suggestive of physical dependence.
- Recreational use and abuse seems to occur more often with pregabalin than gabapentin, often at supratherapeutic dosing for the euphoric effects. Those with opioid use disorders have much higher gabapentin and pregabalin abuse rates.
- Pregabalin is related in structure to gabapentin, which is (so far, according to the DEA) not a controlled substance but is more potent, with faster absorption and greater bioavailability.
- For generalized anxiety disorder, pregabalin appears more effective than placebo, but data comparing it to benzodiazepines are inconsistent.

Fun Fact:

Other drugs related to gabapentin and pregabalin are being studied; Pfizer was developing atagabalin for use in insomnia, but it discontinued development due to disappointing trial results.

Bottom Line:

Try pregabalin in a patient with generalized anxiety disorder who has failed or not tolerated SSRI trials. It can also be helpful for patients struggling to discontinue benzodiazepines.

TOPIRAMATE (Topamax) Fact Sheet [G]

FDA Indications:
Seizure disorders for patients ≥2 years; migraine prophylaxis.

Off-Label Uses:
Alcohol dependence; bipolar disorder; PTSD; binge-eating disorder; obesity.

Dosage Forms:
- **Tablets (G):** 25 mg, 50 mg, 100 mg, 200 mg.
- **Capsules (G):** 15 mg, 25 mg.
- **Capsules, ER (Trokendi XR, Qudexy XR, G):** 25 mg, 50 mg, 100 mg, 150 mg, 200 mg.

Dosage Guidance:
Seizures/migraine: Start 25 mg–50 mg QHS and ↑ by 50 mg/day in weekly increments. Doses used in psychiatry have typically been 50 mg–300 mg/day, divided BID (ER can be given QHS).

Monitoring: Baseline and periodic serum bicarbonate.

Cost: IR: $; ER: $$$$

Side Effects:
- Most common: Somnolence, dizziness, nervousness, ataxia, speech problems, memory difficulties, confusion, anorexia.
- Serious but rare: Decreases in serum bicarbonate (metabolic acidosis) relatively common but usually mild to moderate; more severe cases, including marked reductions to <17 mEq/L, may occur more rarely. Watch for kidney stones, osteomalacia.

Mechanism, Pharmacokinetics, and Drug Interactions:
- Sodium channel blocker.
- Not metabolized, excreted primarily unchanged; t ½: 21 hours (56 hours for XR); mild CYP3A4 inducer.
- Avoid concomitant use with hydrochlorothiazide, which can increase risk for hypokalemia; monitor potassium. Avoid in patients with metabolic acidosis taking concomitant metformin. Additive effects with sedatives or alcohol. Concurrent use with valproic acid may increase risk of hyperammonemia and associated encephalopathy. Higher doses (>200 mg/day) may decrease levels of some drugs, including contraceptives (P450 induction).

Clinical Pearls:
- Many published articles have shown some efficacy in a wide range of disorders, including bipolar disorder, PTSD, alcohol dependence, binge-eating disorder, and obesity.
- Most compelling data is for preventing relapse in alcoholism.
- Some patients may lose weight, but this is not common; greatest decrease in weight seems to occur in heaviest patients (>100 kg). When weight loss occurs, it is often not a large effect (mean of 6 kg) nor is it a sustained effect (patients return to pretreatment weight after 12–18 months).
- A combination of extended release topiramate and phentermine was FDA approved in 2012 for the long-term treatment of obesity as Qsymia (Vivus Pharmaceuticals).

Fun Fact:
Dose-related cognitive effects of topiramate have led some to refer to Topamax as "Dopamax."

Bottom Line:
Topiramate is a reasonable off-label choice for alcohol use disorder. Otherwise, relegate it to the "try when out of other ideas" category.

Sexual Dysfunction Medications

GENERAL PRESCRIBING TIPS

Many psychiatric medications cause sexual dysfunction. Most antidepressants (the main exceptions being bupropion and mirtazapine) cause sexual problems, which can include low libido, anorgasmia, and erectile dysfunction. Antipsychotics often lower libido, whether due to increased prolactin or other unknown factors.

Before jumping to treat the side effect of one medication with another medication, try other potential solutions. You can try decreasing the dose of the offending medication, switching to another medication, adding an "antidote" such as bupropion or mirtazapine in the case of antidepressant-induced effects, or prescribing 2- to 3-day drug holidays.

Assuming none of these strategies has worked, you might want to prescribe one of the medications in this section. Here's one approach.

For males who have erectile dysfunction, prescribe one of the PDE-5 inhibitors, of which there are 4 available options. Sildenafil (Viagra) has the benefit of being well known to patients, which might enhance the placebo effect. Tadalafil (Cialis) has the advantage of a long (up to 36 hours) duration of action. Avanafil (Stendra) works a little more quickly than Viagra—15 minutes as opposed to 30 minutes. Vardenafil (Levitra) is available as a peppermint-flavored orally disintegrating pill—though it has no therapeutic advantages beyond whatever aphrodisiac power peppermint might provide.

For females with low sexual desire, there is one approved medication—flibanserin (Addyi). It doesn't work very well, and it can't be mixed with alcohol, so it's unlikely to become popular. Many believe that its approval was driven more by politics than science.

For both men and women who suffer sexual dysfunction from serotonergic antidepressants, you can try off-label cyproheptadine. It works pretty well sometimes, but other times it doesn't work at all. Adjunctive bupropion or mirtazapine sometimes helps as well.

For men with low testosterone, prescribe . . . testosterone. It will add zip to patients who suffer low libido as a result of low T. However, don't get roped into prescribing this for anyone who asks for it, since there's no evidence it helps men with normal T levels.

Class Warnings for PDE-5 Inhibitors

Avoid concomitant use with nitrates in any form—eg, nitroglycerin, isosorbide dinitrate, amyl nitrite ("poppers").

TABLE 14: Sexual Dysfunction Medications

Generic Name (Brand Name) Year FDA Approved *[G] denotes generic availability*	Relevant FDA Indication(s)	Available Strengths (mg)	Starting Dose (mg)	Usual Dosage Range (starting–max) (mg)	Special Features
Avanafil (Stendra) 2012	Erectile dysfunction	50, 100, 200	100	50–200	More rapid onset (15 minutes); food doesn't affect absorption
Cyproheptadine [G] 1961 Brand name Periactin discontinued; generic only	None	4; 2/5 mL	4	4–12	Sedating; most effective for anorgasmia
Flibanserin (Addyi) 2015	Hypoactive sexual desire disorder in premenopausal women	100	100	100	Can't be combined with alcohol
Sildenafil [G] (Viagra) 1998 Generic only available as 20 mg tablet	Erectile dysfunction	25, 50, 100	25	25–100	Takes 30 minutes; fatty meals decrease absorption
Tadalafil (Cialis) 2003	Erectile dysfunction	2.5, 5, 10, 20	5	5–20	Takes 1 hour, lasts 36 hours; no meal effect
Testosterone	Hypogonadism	Various formulations and dosages; see fact sheet for details			No evidence of beneficial effect in the absence of low T
Vardenafil (Levitra) 2003	Erectile dysfunction	2.5, 5, 10, 20	10	10–20	Works in 30 minutes; fatty meals decrease absorption
Vardenafil ODT (Staxyn) 2010	Erectile dysfunction	10 ODT	10	10	Peppermint flavored

AVANAFIL (Stendra) Fact Sheet

FDA Indications:
Erectile dysfunction.

Dosage Forms:
Tablets: 50 mg, 100 mg, 200 mg.

Dosage Guidance:
- Start 100 mg x1 taken 15 minutes before sexual activity. Max dose 200 mg/dose, up to 1 dose/24 hours.
- May be taken with or without food.

Monitoring: No routine monitoring recommended unless clinical picture warrants.

Cost: $$$$

Side Effects:
- Most common: Headache, nasal congestion, flushing.
- Serious but rare: May cause dose-related impairment of color discrimination. Sudden decrease or loss of hearing has been reported rarely; hearing changes may be accompanied by tinnitus and dizziness. Decreases in blood pressure may occur due to vasodilator effects; concurrent use with alpha-adrenergic antagonists or substantial alcohol consumption may cause symptomatic hypotension. Avoid use with nitrates (see below). Painful erection >6 hours in duration (priapism) may occur rarely.

Mechanism, Pharmacokinetics, and Drug Interactions:
- Phosphodiesterase type 5 (PDE-5) inhibitor.
- Metabolized primarily through CYP3A4, also 2C9/19 to a lesser degree; t ½: 5 hours.
- Avoid concomitant use with nitrates in any form (eg, nitroglycerin, isosorbide dinitrate, amyl nitrite "poppers"). Use with caution in patients taking alpha-adrenergic blockers; may cause symptomatic hypotension (maximum of 50 mg in 24 hours). Use with caution in patients taking strong CYP3A4 inhibitors, which may increase or extend effects of avanafil (maximum of 50 mg in 24 hours).

Clinical Pearls:
Onset of effect is usually 15–30 minutes after a dose (and not affected by meals). About two-thirds of men will have therapeutic effect within 15 minutes. Usual duration is approximately 2 hours.

Fun Fact:
Avanafil was initially approved with the recommendation to take it 30 minutes before sexual activity. Its manufacturer decided it was tough to compete with blockbusters like Viagra and Cialis without some sort of competitive edge, so it presented some data to the FDA and had the dosing changed to "as early as approximately 15 minutes before sexual activity." Spontaneity became the hallmark of the drug's marketing campaign, with taglines like "This time, he was ready before dessert."

Bottom Line:
Avanafil is the newest PDE-5 inhibitor to come to market. Its potential advantage is a somewhat faster onset than any of the other ED drugs.

CYPROHEPTADINE Fact Sheet [G]

FDA Indications:
Allergic rhinitis; urticaria.

Off-Label Uses:
Antidepressant-induced sexual dysfunction; anorexia and bulimia nervosa; appetite stimulant; acute management of serotonin syndrome.

Dosage Forms:
- **Tablets (G):** 4 mg (scored).
- **Syrup (G):** 2 mg/5 mL syrup.

Dosage Guidance:
Take 4 mg–12 mg 1–2 hours before sexual activity.

Monitoring: No routine monitoring recommended unless clinical picture warrants.

Cost: $

Side Effects:
Most common: Sedation, confusion, weight gain, anticholinergic effects, potential reversal of antidepressant therapeutic effect.

Mechanism, Pharmacokinetics, and Drug Interactions:
- Histamine H1 receptor antagonist with mild antiserotonergic effects.
- Metabolized primarily through hepatic glucuronidation via UGT1A; t ½: 16 hours.
- Avoid concomitant use with MAOIs. Additive effects with other sedating agents.

Clinical Pearls:
- Appears to work best for anorgasmia. Average effective dose in one study was 8.6 mg.
- Excessive sedation may impede therapeutic efficacy in some patients.

Fun Facts:
Cyproheptadine's antagonistic effects at serotonin receptors have been shown to be useful as part of the management of serotonin syndrome. It's been used to counteract the more rarely occurring serotonergic side effects of serotonergic antidepressants, such as sweating and vivid dreams. It is also the most commonly used appetite stimulant for cats.

Bottom Line:
Cyproheptadine is sometimes effective in reversing SSRI-induced anorgasmia, but with continued use it could interfere with antidepressant efficacy. As-needed occasional use is the best strategy.

FLIBANSERIN (Addyi) Fact Sheet

FDA Indications:
Hypoactive sexual desire disorder in premenopausal women.

Dosage Forms:
Tablets: 100 mg.

Dosage Guidance:
Start and continue 100 mg QHS; taking during the daytime may increase risk of hypotension, syncope, and CNS depression. Discontinue after 8 weeks if no improvement.

Monitoring: No routine monitoring recommended unless clinical picture warrants.

Cost: $$$$$

Side Effects:
- Most common: Dizziness, somnolence, nausea, fatigue, insomnia, dry mouth.
- Serious but rare: May have potential to cause severe hypotension or syncope.

Mechanism, Pharmacokinetics, and Drug Interactions:
- Mixed agonist-antagonist on postsynaptic serotonergic receptors with 5-HT1A agonist and 5-HT2A antagonist effects.
- Metabolized primarily through CYP3A4 and to a lesser extent, 2C19; t ½: 11 hours.
- Avoid concomitant use with alcohol, with CYP3A4 inhibitors, or in patients with hepatic impairment as there may be an increased risk for hypotension and syncope.

Clinical Pearls:
- Addyi has not been studied in postmenopausal women or men.
- Addyi does not enhance sexual performance; rather, it increases interest.
- While studies of Viagra show around 80% of men improving (50%–60% more than placebo), only 8%–13% more women on flibanserin had benefits over placebo.
- Addyi is available only through a restricted program called the Addyi REMS Program because of the increased risk of severe hypotension and syncope due to an interaction between Addyi and alcohol (prescribers must be enrolled, trained, and certified).

Fun Fact:
Based on mediocre efficacy data, Dr. Carlat has made the analogy that "if Viagra is a Starbucks triple espresso, flibanserin is a Dixie cup of cafeteria coffee."

Bottom Line:
This "pink Viagra" is a mildly effective medication with potentially significant side effects. Until we have more data and experience, consider cautiously prescribing it to women who might benefit from it.

SILDENAFIL (Viagra) Fact Sheet [G]

FDA Indications:
Erectile dysfunction; pulmonary arterial hypertension (Revatio brand name).

Dosage Forms:
Tablets: 25 mg, 50 mg, 100 mg.

Dosage Guidance:
Start 50 mg x1 (25 mg if >65 years old or with CYP3A4 inhibitors) 30 minutes–4 hours before sexual activity. Max 100 mg/dose and 1 dose/day. Avoid taking with a high-fat meal.

Monitoring: No routine monitoring recommended unless clinical picture warrants.

Cost: $

Side Effects:
- Most common: Headache, dyspepsia/heartburn, flushing.
- Serious but rare: May cause dose-related impairment of color discrimination. Sudden decrease or loss of hearing has been reported rarely; hearing changes may be accompanied by tinnitus and dizziness. Decreases in blood pressure may occur due to vasodilator effects; concurrent use with alpha-adrenergic antagonists or substantial alcohol consumption may cause symptomatic hypotension. Avoid use with nitrates (see below). Painful erection >6 hours in duration (priapism) may occur rarely.

Mechanism, Pharmacokinetics, and Drug Interactions:
- Phosphodiesterase type 5 (PDE-5) inhibitor.
- Metabolized primarily through CYP3A4 and to a lesser extent, 2C9; t ½: 4 hours.
- Avoid concomitant use with nitrates in any form (eg, nitroglycerin, isosorbide dinitrate, amyl nitrite "poppers"). Use with caution in patients taking alpha-adrenergic blockers; may cause symptomatic hypotension (use 25 mg dose). Use with caution in patients taking strong CYP3A4 inhibitors, which may increase or extend effects of sildenafil (maximum of 25 mg in 48 hours).

Clinical Pearl:
Onset of effect is usually 15–20 minutes after a dose (but may be delayed 60 minutes by a high-fat meal), and usual duration is approximately 2 hours.

Fun Fact:
Sildenafil has been used recreationally. Some users mix it with MDMA (ecstasy) to counteract the erectile dysfunction MDMA can cause; this combination is known as "sextasy."

Bottom Line:
Of the agents in this class, sildenafil has the best evidence and longest track record.

TADALAFIL (Cialis) Fact Sheet

FDA Indications:
Erectile dysfunction; benign prostatic hyperplasia; pulmonary arterial hypertension (Adcirca brand name).

Dosage Forms:
Tablets: 2.5 mg, 5 mg, 10 mg, 20 mg.

Dosage Guidance:
- PRN dosing: Start 10 mg x1, 30–60 minutes prior to sexual activity; adjust dose to 5 mg–20 mg based on response. Max 20 mg/dose and 1 dose/24 hours.
- Daily dosing: Start 2.5 mg QD; may increase to max of 5 mg QD based on response.

Monitoring: No routine monitoring recommended unless clinical picture warrants.

Cost: $$$$

Side Effects:
- Most common: Headache, dyspepsia/nausea, flushing, back pain, muscle aches.
- Serious but rare: May cause dose-related impairment of color discrimination. Sudden decrease or loss of hearing has been reported rarely; hearing changes may be accompanied by tinnitus and dizziness. Decreases in blood pressure may occur due to vasodilator effects; concurrent use with alpha-adrenergic antagonists or substantial alcohol consumption may cause symptomatic hypotension. Avoid use with nitrates (see below). Painful erection >6 hours in duration (priapism) may occur rarely.

Mechanism, Pharmacokinetics, and Drug Interactions:
- Phosphodiesterase type 5 (PDE-5) inhibitor.
- Metabolized primarily through CYP3A4; t ½: 15–17.5 hours.
- Avoid concomitant use with nitrates in any form (eg, nitroglycerin, isosorbide dinitrate, amyl nitrite "poppers"). Use with caution in patients taking alpha-adrenergic blockers; may cause symptomatic hypotension (use lower tadalafil dose). Use with caution in patients taking strong CYP3A4 inhibitors, which may increase or extend effects of tadalafil (maximum of 10 mg/dose and 1 dose/72 hours with PRN dosing or 2.5 mg/day with daily dosing).

Clinical Pearls:
- Onset of effect of tadalafil is usually within 1 hour, and its effects may last 36 hours.
- Daily tadalafil has the advantage of allowing users to always be "ready," but it can also cause daily side effects.

Fun Fact:
Cialis' 36-hour effectiveness earned it the nickname "the weekend pill."

Bottom Line:
We have fewer data for tadalafil in the psychiatric setting; however, compared to other agents in the class, its long duration of action may improve spontaneity, and the lack of interaction with meals may offer advantages.

TESTOSTERONE (various) Fact Sheet [G]

FDA Indications:
Hypogonadism.

Dosage Forms:
- **Capsules (Android):** 10 mg methyltestosterone.
- **Buccal ER tablet (Striant):** 30 mg.
- **Topical gel (AndroGel, Androderm, others):** 1%, 2%.
- **Long-acting depot injection (Depo-Testosterone, [G]):** 100 mg/mL, 200 mg/mL.

Dosage Guidance:
- Dosing varies from daily dosing of oral, buccal, and topical agents to Q2–4 week or Q3–6 month dosing of injectable formulations.
- Schedule III controlled substance.

Monitoring: Hematocrit, bone density, liver function tests.

Cost: Capsule: $$$$$; buccal: $$$$$; gel: $$$$; depot injectable: $

Side Effects:
- Most common: Nausea, headache, insomnia, anxiety, acne, water and electrolyte retention, local effects (eg, gum irritation with buccal formulation, application site irritation with gel, injection site pain with injectables).
- Serious but rare: Thromboembolic events (DVT, PE), myocardial infarction, stroke, worsening BPH, risk of prostate cancer.

Mechanism, Pharmacokinetics, and Drug Interactions:
- Anabolic and andronergic testosterone receptor agonist.
- Metabolized primarily through liver (non-CYP450); t ½: Varies.

Clinical Pearls:
- Hypogonadism may play a significant role in erectile dysfunction (ED), and a threshold level of testosterone may be necessary for normal erectile function. However, testosterone levels needed for normal sexual function vary widely; some men may have normal function even with age-adjusted lower normal range levels. Testosterone replacement may be appropriate when both clinical symptoms and biochemical evidence of hypogonadism exist.
- Available data indicate that all testosterone products may be equally effective and associated with similar side effect profiles.

Fun Fact:
Stephen Braun, a medical writer, described how he was funded by Abbott Pharmaceuticals to help write a "consensus panel" statement for a physician's organization. Two of his paragraphs casting doubt on the dangers of low testosterone were deleted from the final document (Braun S, *JAMA Internal Medicine* 2013;173(15):1458–1460).

Bottom Line:
Successful marketing has convinced the public that "low T" is a public health scourge, leading to over-prescribing of testosterone for patients who don't need it. Prescribe it only for men with demonstrably low testosterone levels and accompanying symptoms.

VARDENAFIL (Levitra) Fact Sheet

FDA Indications:
Erectile dysfunction.

Dosage Forms:
- **Tablets:** 2.5 mg, 5 mg, 10 mg, 20 mg.
- **Orally disintegrating tablets (Staxyn):** 10 mg.

Dosage Guidance:
- Start 10 mg x1, 1 hour prior to sexual activity (5 mg if >65 years old). Max 20 mg/dose and 1 dose/day.
- ODT (Staxyn): Start 10 mg x1, 1 hour prior to sexual activity. Max 10 mg/day.
- Taking with a high-fat meal may decrease serum vardenafil levels by as much as 50%.

Monitoring: No routine monitoring recommended unless clinical picture warrants.

Cost: $$$$$

Side Effects:
- Most common: Flushing, headache, nasal congestion, heartburn.
- Serious but rare: May cause dose-related impairment of color discrimination. Sudden decrease or loss of hearing has been reported rarely; hearing changes may be accompanied by tinnitus and dizziness. Decreases in blood pressure may occur due to vasodilator effects; concurrent use with alpha-adrenergic antagonists or substantial alcohol consumption may cause symptomatic hypotension. Avoid use with nitrates (see below). Painful erection >6 hours in duration (priapism) may occur rarely.

Mechanism, Pharmacokinetics, and Drug Interactions:
- Phosphodiesterase type 5 (PDE-5) inhibitor.
- Metabolized primarily through CYP3A4 and to a lesser extent, 2C9; t ½: 4–5 hours.
- Avoid concomitant use with nitrates in any form (eg, nitroglycerin, isosorbide dinitrate, amyl nitrite "poppers"). Use with caution in patients taking alpha-blockers; may cause symptomatic hypotension (use 5 mg dose). Use with caution in patients taking strong CYP3A4 inhibitors, which may increase or extend effects of vardenafil (maximum of 2.5 mg/day).

Clinical Pearl:
Usual onset of effect of vardenafil is within 1 hour of a dose; effects usually last 2 hours.

Fun Fact:
Staxyn, the orally disintegrating tablet form of vardenafil, is peppermint flavored.

Bottom Line:
Vardenafil doesn't offer any benefits compared to sildenafil, which has more data in the psychiatric setting and more clinical experience.

Side Effect Management

GENERAL MANAGEMENT TIPS

If you're like most psychiatrists, you probably severely underestimate the number of side effects your patients are experiencing. According to one survey, patients on antidepressants reported *20 times* more side effects than were actually recorded by their psychiatrists (Zimmerman M et al, *J Clin Psychiatry* 2010;71(4):484–490).

Sometimes we don't ask about side effects because we wouldn't know what to do about them. In order to help you expand your side effect battling arsenal, we have created this new side effect management section for the 4th edition of the *Medication Fact Book.* We've included 16 fact sheets covering some of the most common side effects you are likely to encounter in your patients. We had to pick and choose which ones to include, so if there are important symptoms that are missing, please let us know so we can add them to the next edition.

In addition to the side effect management sheets, we've included 6 regular medication fact sheets on agents that we use primarily to treat side effects. These include amantadine, benztropine, and trihexyphenidyl for extrapyramidal symptoms of antipsychotics; deutetrabenazine and valbenazine for tardive dyskinesia; and metformin for weight gain caused by psychotropic drugs.

Here's a quick orientation to the side effect fact sheet format:

- *Characteristics:* We describe what the side effect feels like for patients and how you can recognize it.
- *Meds That Cause It:* These are the medications that are most likely to cause the side effect in question. We include only psychotropics in this list.
- *Mechanism:* Although we usually don't know exactly how psychotropics cause most side effects, we posit mechanisms that seem to be most popular with experts.
- *General Management:* This refers to everything other than prescribing specific antidotes. Included here are things like watchful waiting, reducing the dose, switching to a different medication, shifting the timing of the dose (usually to bedtime), taking with food, and so on. Mostly these are commonsense interventions, which you should try before prescribing a new anti–side effect medication.
- *First-Line Medications:* In some cases, most experts agree on a few medications that are most likely to be effective for managing specific side effects. That said, since there are very few clinical trials testing meds for side effects, judgments about what qualifies as a first-line vs a second-line medication are fallible, and we won't be offended if you disagree.
- *Second-Line Medications:* This section is reserved for the various nostrums—drugs that have been tried by various people and might work. Often you would resort to these only out of desperation.
- *Clinical Pearls:* Hard-won wisdom from the trenches.
- *Fun Fact:* Sometimes entertaining, sometimes intriguing . . . and sometimes just present.

A note on information sources: It's not easy to find reliable information on side effect management. There are very few well-designed clinical trials on such uses, meaning that we must rely on uncontrolled trials, small case series, anecdotes, or simply expert opinion. In doing research for the symptom fact sheets in this section, we relied primarily on the following three sources, supplemented by various articles and our own clinical experiences:

- Annamalai A, Medical Management of Psychotropic Side Effects. New York, NY: Springer Publishing; 2017.
- Goldberg JF and Ernst CL, Managing the Side Effects of Psychotropic Medications. Arlington, VA: American Psychiatric Association; 2012.
- Mago R, Side Effects of Psychiatric Medications. Createspace Independent Pub; 2014.

AMANTADINE (Gocovri, Symmetrel) Fact Sheet [G]

FDA Indications:
Drug-induced extrapyramidal symptoms (EPS); Parkinson's disease; influenza A (though CDC recommends against use due to resistance).

Off-Label Uses:
ADHD; enuresis; treatment-resistant depression; OCD.

Dosage Forms:
- **Capsules (G):** 100 mg.
- **Tablets (G):** 100 mg.
- **Oral solution (G):** 50 mg/5 mL.
- **ER capsules (Gocovri):** 68.5 mg, 137 mg.

Dosage Guidance:
- IR: Start 100 mg BID. Max 300 mg/day.
- ER: Start 137 mg QHS; increase after 1 week to usual and max dose of 274 mg QHS.

Monitoring: No routine monitoring recommended unless clinical picture warrants.

Cost: $; ER: $$$$$

Side Effects:
- Most common: Nausea, dizziness, orthostatic hypotension, insomnia, blurred vision, constipation, dry mouth.
- Serious but rare: Rare cases of intense urges to gamble, spend money, or have sex reported.

Mechanism, Pharmacokinetics, and Drug Interactions:
- Weak NMDA antagonist and potentiates dopaminergic neurons. Antiviral (inhibits replication of influenza A virus).
- Not metabolized; excreted primarily through kidneys; t ½: 17 hours.
- Minimal clinically significant drug interactions.

Clinical Pearls:
- Because of dopaminergic effects, theoretically amantadine could worsen psychosis. At doses typically used to manage EPS, though, this doesn't generally happen.
- Typically used when anticholinergic side effects of other anti-EPS medications (benztropine, trihexyphenidyl) are intolerable.
- Adjust dose in elderly patients or those with impaired renal function.
- Gocovri is a high-dose extended release once-daily version of amantadine, approved for treatment of dyskinesia in Parkinson's patients taking levodopa. It's estimated to cost patients $10,000–$30,000 per year.

Fun Fact:
Memantine (Namenda), an NMDA antagonist used in dementia, is an analogue of amantadine.

Bottom Line:
In older patients who develop EPS, particularly Parkinsonian symptoms, amantadine may be a good alternative with fewer anticholinergic side effects.

BENZTROPINE (Cogentin) Fact Sheet [G]

FDA Indications:

Drug-induced extrapyramidal symptoms (EPS); Parkinson's disease.

Off-Label Uses:

Sialorrhea (excessive salivation); hyperhidrosis (excessive sweating).

Dosage Forms:

- **Tablets (G):** 0.5 mg, 1 mg, 2 mg.
- **Injectable:** 1 mg/mL.

Dosage Guidance:

- Start 1 mg BID; max 3 mg BID. May be taken once daily at bedtime.
- For acute dystonic reactions, use 1 mg–2 mg IM x 1 and continue with oral, as above, to prevent recurrence.

Monitoring: No routine monitoring recommended unless clinical picture warrants.

Cost: $

Side Effects:

- Most common: Dry mouth, blurred vision, constipation, urinary retention, sedation.
- Serious but rare: In those at risk (elderly patients), may cause confusion or delirium; may worsen angle-closure glaucoma.

Mechanism, Pharmacokinetics, and Drug Interactions:

- Anticholinergic, antihistaminergic.
- Metabolized primarily through liver via unknown P450; t ½: 12–24 hours.
- Minimal clinically significant drug interactions; avoid combining with other anticholinergic agents due to additive effects.

Clinical Pearls:

If starting a patient on a high-potency antipsychotic such as haloperidol or risperidone, some clinicians will start benztropine prophylactically to prevent EPS. If you do so, consider taper and withdrawal of benztropine after 1–2 weeks to see if it's really needed.

Fun Fact:

Veterinarians use benztropine to treat priapism in stallions.

Bottom Line:

Go-to agent for treating and preventing antipsychotic-induced EPS.

DEUTETRABENAZINE (Austedo) Fact Sheet

FDA Indications:
Tardive dyskinesia (TD); Huntington's chorea.

Off-Label Uses:
Tourette's and other tic disorders.

Dosage Forms:
Tablets: 6 mg, 9 mg, 12 mg.

Dosage Guidance:
Start 6 mg BID with food. Titrate at weekly intervals by 6 mg/day; increase to maximum dose of 48 mg/day with food (doses ≥12 mg/day should be divided BID).

Monitoring: ECG if cardiac disease.

Cost: $$$$$

Side Effects:
- Most common: Sedation, somnolence, fatigue, diarrhea.
- Serious but rare: QT interval prolongation; caution in those with increased risk (congenital long QT syndrome, electrolyte disturbances, poor 2D6 metabolizers, concomitant 2D6 inhibitors).

Mechanism, Pharmacokinetics, and Drug Interactions:
- Reversible inhibitor of vesicular monoamine transporter 2 (VMAT2). This prevents VMAT2 from transporting dopamine back into the neuron, so that it remains in the synaptic space and is vulnerable to metabolism, ultimately leading to less dopamine being around. This treats TD symptoms, which are likely caused by hypersensitivity to dopamine.
- Metabolized primarily by CYP450 2D6; t ½: 9–10 hours.
- Avoid MAOIs. Decrease deutetrabenazine dose in presence of 2D6 inhibitors or poor metabolizers.

Clinical Pearls:
- Deutetrabenazine is a deuterated form of tetrabenazine (Xenazine), a similar VMAT2 inhibitor, which is approved for treatment of Huntington's chorea.
- Increased depression and suicidality have been reported with tetrabenazine. Paucity of long-term data with deutetrabenazine makes it difficult to determine whether it will pose these concerns as well.
- A one-year course costs over $60,000.

Fun Fact:
Chemistry course refresher! Deuterated drugs are created by replacing one or more of the hydrogen atoms of the drug molecule by deuterium. This may significantly slow drug metabolism, resulting in a longer half-life of the drug.

Bottom Line:
It's best to prevent TD from developing in the first place. Use the AIMS (Abnormal Involuntary Movement Scale) to monitor your patients, and decrease doses or switch medications in patients who have signs of TD. If you must treat the TD, consider generic tetrabenazine first before the incredibly expensive deutetrabenazine or valbenazine. Tetrabenazine is somewhat cheaper, but still expensive, and while not FDA approved for TD, it probably works just as well. Its downside is a black box warning about suicidality.

METFORMIN (Glucophage) Fact Sheet [G]

FDA Indications:

Diabetes mellitus, type 2.

Off-Label Uses:

Weight management (eg, for those with weight gain due to antipsychotics); polycystic ovary syndrome; prediabetes; female infertility.

Dosage Forms:

- **Tablets (G):** 500 mg, 850 mg, 1000 mg.
- **ER tablets (G):** 500 mg, 750 mg, 1000 mg.

Dosage Guidance:

- IR: Start 500 mg BID; ↑ by 500 mg/day increments weekly; max 2250 mg/day.
- ER: Start 500 mg QPM; ↑ by 500 mg/day increments weekly; max 2000 mg/day.

Monitoring: No routine monitoring recommended unless clinical picture warrants.

Cost: $

Side Effects:

- Most common: Diarrhea, nausea, abdominal bloating, flatulence and discomfort.
- Serious but rare: Rare cases of lactic acidosis reported.

Mechanism, Pharmacokinetics, and Drug Interactions:

- Decreases glucose production by liver and increases insulin sensitivity.
- Not metabolized; excreted primarily through kidneys; t ½: 4–9 hours.
- Minimal clinically significant drug interactions.

Clinical Pearls:

- In psychiatry, metformin is used primarily to prevent or reverse weight gain in patients taking certain antipsychotic medications.
- A recent meta-analysis of 12 studies, representing a total of 743 patients, found metformin use resulted in more weight loss (an average of about 7 pounds) and BMI reduction than placebo in patients taking antipsychotics (de Silva VA et al, *BMC Psychiatry* 2016;16:341).
- Another review of patients with schizophrenia who were treated with antipsychotics found metformin also improved insulin resistance and decreased lipids (Mizuno Y et al, *Schizophrenia Bulletin* 2014;40(6):1385–1403).

Fun Fact:

Metformin was introduced in the US in 1995, but it's been in use in France since 1957.

Bottom Line:

Preventing weight gain is still the best approach, but metformin is a safe and moderately effective agent to counteract the weight gain caused by antipsychotics like clozapine and olanzapine.

TRIHEXYPHENIDYL (Artane) Fact Sheet [G]

FDA Indications:

Drug-induced extrapyramidal symptoms (EPS); Parkinson's disease.

Off-Label Uses:

Sialorrhea (excessive salivation); hyperhidrosis (excessive sweating).

Dosage Forms:

- **Tablets (G):** 2 mg, 5 mg.
- **Oral solution:** 2 mg/5 mL.

Dosage Guidance:

Start 2 mg QD; ↑ by 2 mg/day every 3–5 days, up to 5 mg TID.

Monitoring: No routine monitoring recommended unless clinical picture warrants.

Cost: $

Side Effects:

- Most common: Dry mouth, blurred vision, constipation, urinary retention, sedation.
- Serious but rare: In those at risk (elderly patients), may cause confusion or delirium; may worsen angle-closure glaucoma.

Mechanism, Pharmacokinetics, and Drug Interactions:

- Anticholinergic, antihistaminergic.
- Metabolized primarily through liver via unknown P450; t ½: 3–4 hours.
- Minimal clinically significant drug interactions; avoid combining with other anticholinergic agents due to additive effects.

Clinical Pearls:

If starting a patient on a high-potency antipsychotic such as haloperidol or risperidone, some clinicians will start trihexyphenidyl prophylactically to prevent EPS. If you do so, consider taper and withdrawal of trihexyphenidyl after 1–2 weeks to see if it's really needed.

Fun Fact:

There have been many reports of recreational use of trihexyphenidyl over the years: by Iraqi soldiers and police to relieve combat stress, as a more intense substitute for LSD in the 1960s, and by the late Oliver Sacks, who reportedly took 20 trihexyphenidyl pills and hallucinated an entire conversation with friends (check out his book, *Hallucinations*, to read about his experimentation with a range of drugs).

Bottom Line:

Less favored than benztropine because it must be dosed TID and is only available in oral formulations. Use as a second-line option.

VALBENAZINE (Ingrezza) Fact Sheet

FDA Indications:
Tardive dyskinesia (TD).

Off-Label Uses:
Tourette's and other tic disorders; Huntington's chorea.

Dosage Forms:
Capsules: 40 mg.

Dosage Guidance:
Start 40 mg once daily. After one week, increase to usual dose of 80 mg once daily.

Monitoring: ECG if cardiac disease.

Cost: $$$$$

Side Effects:
- Most common: Sedation, somnolence, akathisia, restlessness.
- Serious but rare: QT interval prolongation; caution in those with increased risk (congenital long QT syndrome, electrolyte disturbances, poor 2D6 metabolizers, concomitant 2D6 or 3A4 inhibitors).

Mechanism, Pharmacokinetics, and Drug Interactions:
- Reversible inhibitor of vesicular monoamine transporter 2 (VMAT2). This prevents VMAT2 from transporting dopamine back into the neuron, so that it remains in the synaptic space and is vulnerable to metabolism, ultimately leading to less dopamine being around. This treats TD symptoms, which are likely caused by hypersensitivity to dopamine.
- Metabolized by CYP450 2D6 and 3A4 (primary); t ½: 15–22 hours.
- Avoid MAOIs. Decrease valbenazine dose in presence of 2D6 or 3A4 inhibitors.

Clinical Pearls:
- Clinical trials of valbenazine for TD found an impressive 40% response rate (meaning a 50% improvement in TD symptoms) vs a 9% response rate for patients taking placebo.
- Increased depression and suicidality have been reported with use of a similar VMAT2 inhibitor, tetrabenazine (Xenazine, used for Huntington's chorea). Paucity of long-term data with valbenazine makes it difficult to determine whether this will be of concern with valbenazine as well.
- A one-year course costs over $63,000.

Fun Fact:
Reserpine, an antihypertensive and antipsychotic used in the 1950s, was a VMAT1/VMAT2 inhibitor. Cases of depression reported with its use led to the monoamine hypothesis of depression.

Bottom Line:
It's best to prevent TD from developing in the first place. Use the AIMS (Abnormal Involuntary Movement Scale) to monitor your patients, and decrease doses or switch medications in patients who have signs of TD. If you must treat the TD, you can consider valbenazine. But it's incredibly expensive, and there are generic VMAT2 inhibitors on the market, such as tetrabenazine. Tetrabenazine is somewhat cheaper, but still expensive, and while not FDA approved for TD, it probably works just as well. Its downside is a black box warning about suicidality.

Akathisia

Characteristics: A sense of restlessness, causing the patient to appear fidgety, to have difficulty sitting still, and to rock from one leg to the other while standing. It can present as an inner sense of restlessness without obvious movement. Can lead to agitation and even suicidal ideation.

Meds That Cause It: Antipsychotics, especially high-potency typical agents, but several atypical agents may also cause it (aripiprazole, asenapine, brexpiprazole, cariprazine, lurasidone, paliperidone, risperidone). Occasionally SSRIs and buspirone.

Mechanism: D2 blockade.

General Management:

- Reduce dose.
- Switch to lower-potency agent or different atypical agent.

First-Line Medications:

- Propranolol. Start 10 mg BID; can go up to 30 mg–90 mg daily in two or three divided doses. SE: Dizziness, fatigue, syncope, low BP.
- Inderal LA. Long-acting version of propranolol that can be dosed once a day. 60 mg–80 mg daily.
- Benzodiazepines. Any of them will work (eg, lorazepam 0.5 mg to 1 mg BID). Dosed at the equivalent of diazepam 10 mg BID or more frequently as needed.

Second-Line Medications:

- Benztropine 1 mg BID.
- Cyproheptadine 8 mg–16 mg/day.
- Amantadine 100 mg–200 mg BID.
- Clonidine 0.2 mg–0.8 mg/day.
- Gabapentin 1200 mg/day.
- Trazodone 100 mg/day.
- Mirtazapine 15 mg/day.

Clinical Pearls:

- May manifest in a number of ways, such as pacing, inability to sit still, crossing and uncrossing one's legs, rocking back and forth, or other purposeless repetitive motions; patients may complain of crawling feeling under skin or "shocks."
- Don't mistake akathisia with agitation due to the underlying psychiatric disorder—you might make the mistake of increasing the antipsychotic, thus worsening the akathisia.
- Risk factors include high dose, high-potency antipsychotics, and rapid dose escalation; use of caffeine, other stimulants, or illicit drugs may also exacerbate akathisia.
- May appear within first few hours of antipsychotic exposure, but usually takes days to weeks to appear.
- Can occur in a tardive form, with symptoms lasting for greater than 6 months after discontinuation of the offending agent.
- Clozapine, quetiapine, and lurasidone cause no more akathisia than placebo.

Fun Fact:

Akathisia is from the Greek *a-kathisis*, "no sitting." The English word "cathedral" is from the same root: *Kathedra* is a bishop's seat or throne, while a cathedral is a church in which the bishop's seat is placed.

Bruxism

Characteristics: Involuntary grinding of teeth, which especially occurs during sleep, but can also occur in the daytime. In 5% of cases this can cause severe health problems, such as destruction of tooth structure, temporomandibular joint dysfunction, myofascial pain, and sleep disturbances.

Meds That Cause It: A variety of medications, including antidepressants (especially SSRIs and the SNRI venlafaxine), psychostimulants, and antipsychotics; drugs of abuse such as methamphetamine, cocaine, and ecstasy.

Mechanism: Unclear, but likely involves central dopaminergic and serotonergic systems.

General Management:

- Reduce dose or switch medication.
- Dental guards worn at night.
- Treat anxiety, which worsens bruxism.
- Decrease or stop smoking tobacco.

First-Line Medications:

- Buspirone (BuSpar) 10 mg BID or TID.

Second-Line Medications:

- Benzodiazepines, such as clonazepam 0.5 mg–1 mg at bedtime.
- Gabapentin (Neurontin) 300 mg QD.

Clinical Pearls:

- Frequency of bruxism varies from day to day, but symptoms are usually induced or worsened by anxiety and stress.
- Watching and waiting may be indicated as spontaneous remission can occur after 1 month.
- Botulinim toxin (botox) injections into the masseter muscle are effective for persistent bruxism.
- Risk factors include obstructive sleep apnea and parasomnias, anxiety, heavy alcohol use, loud snoring, caffeine intake, smoking, and other psychiatric and neurologic disorders.

Fun Fact:

People with bruxism are referred to as "bruxists" or "bruxers."

Constipation

Characteristics: Straining to have bowel movements, often with hard stools, and a sensation of incomplete evacuation. Not necessarily infrequent stools—patients may have a BM every day, but if they strain, they are constipated.

Meds That Cause It: Antipsychotics (especially clozapine and olanzapine, but all can cause it); antidepressants, including SSRIs (particularly paroxetine), SNRIs, mirtazapine, tricyclics, benztropine, antihistamines (eg, diphenhydramine), opiates.

Mechanism: Usually due to anticholinergic effects, which lead to decrease in bowel motility.

General Management:

- Decrease dose or switch agents.
- Increase fluid intake.
- Increase dietary fiber (cereals, fruits, bran) and eat prunes.
- Increase physical activity.

First-Line Medications:

- Bulk-forming laxative (SE: Gas, bloating):
  - Psyllium (Metamucil) or methylcellulose (Citrucel), 1 tablespoon 3 times daily.
- Stool softener (SE: Diarrhea):
  - Docusate sodium (Colace) 100 mg–250 mg twice daily.

Second-Line Medications:

- Osmotic laxatives (SE: Bloating, gas, watery stools):
  - Lactulose 15 mL–30 mL daily or every other day.
  - Polyethylene glycol solution (MiraLax) 8 g–34 g in 8 oz. fluid.
  - Magnesium citrate 150 mL–300 mL daily.
- Stimulant laxatives (SE: Diarrhea, cramps):
  - Sennosides (Ex-Lax, Senokot), available in different formulations.
  - Bisacodyl (Dulcolax) 5 mg–30 mg daily, available as suppository.
  - Milk of magnesia (magnesium hydroxide), available in both chewable tablet and liquid form.

Clinical Pearls:

Constipation can be caused by various illnesses, including irritable bowel syndrome (usually diarrhea interspersed with constipation), hypothyroidism, and colon cancer (red flags include blood in stool and weight loss).

Fun Fact:

According to a crossover trial of 40 patients, prunes worked better than psyllium, producing more spontaneous BMs (3.5 vs 2.8 per week) and better stool consistency (Attaluri A, *Aliment Pharmacol Ther* 2011;33(7):822).

Dry Mouth (Xerostomia)

Characteristics: An uncomfortable sensation of dryness due to diminished saliva; can lead to dental caries, because saliva has an antibacterial effect. Can also cause decreased taste and inflammation of gums.

Meds That Cause It: Most psychotropic meds, especially antipsychotics, antidepressants (including SSRIs), lithium, psychostimulants, and medications used to treat or prevent EPS (benztropine, diphenhydramine, trihexyphenidyl).

Mechanism: Anticholinergic and other effects.

General Management:

- Encourage aggressive oral hygiene, including more frequent dental cleanings.
- Chew sugarless gum to stimulate saliva production (especially gum containing xylitol, which can also reduce dental caries).
- Sip water frequently.
- Suck on ice chips.

First-Line Medications:

- Biotene line of products, OTC (most contain lubricants and humectants to "seal in" moisture):
  - Biotene gum, use as needed.
  - Biotene toothpaste, use as with any toothpaste.
  - Biotene oral rinse (mouthwash), rinse up to 5 times per day.
  - Biotene Oral Balance Gel, use 1 inch on tongue as needed (comes out of a tube).
  - Biotene moisturizing mouth spray, spray on tongue as needed.
- Many saliva substitutes are available, such as Oralube saliva substitute, Oasis mouth spray, and others. No studies have demonstrated superiority of any single brand.

Second-Line Medications:

- Pro-cholinergic drugs:
  - Pilocarpine 5 mg–10 mg 2 or 3 times daily (SE: Sweating, congestion, diarrhea; start with 2.5 mg test dose to ensure tolerability).
  - Cevimeline 30 mg up to 3 times daily.

Clinical Pearls:

- Caffeine can worsen dry mouth, so recommend decreasing caffeine use.
- Don't shy away from trying pro-cholinergic drugs—some patients prefer them over having to constantly use saliva substitute products.

Fun Fact:

Medications are often blamed, particularly in older patients, but aging itself is a common cause of dry mouth.

Dystonia

Characteristics: Involuntary contractions of muscles due to some antipsychotics. Can include torticollis (twisting neck), opisthotonos (arching spine or neck), oculogyric crisis (eyes rolling back), and trismus (jaw clenching). Rare but serious is tongue swelling, which can block the airway or cause choking when eating.

Meds That Cause It: Antipsychotics, especially high-potency typical antipsychotics. May rarely occur with atypical antipsychotics.

Mechanism: D2 blockade.

First-Line Medications: (give these IM or IV if dystonia is severe)

- Benztropine, 1 mg–2 mg once or twice per day (SE: Dry mouth, blurred vision, constipation, urinary retention, and cognitive changes).
- Diphenhydramine, 50 mg/day.
- If dystonia is severe, stop the offending drug, and give either of the above agents IM or IV once or twice to stop the dystonia. Then prescribe 2–3 days of the oral version to prevent another episode.

Second-Line Medications:

- Benzodiazepines (especially diazepam 5 mg–10 mg).
- Amantadine 100 mg–200 mg BID (no injectable available).
- Trihexyphenidyl 1 mg–2 mg TID (no injectable available).

Clinical Pearls:

- Earliest of the EPS, with an onset of hours to days after antipsychotic is started or dose is increased; 90% of reactions occur within first 5 days.
- Risk factors include young male patients, high-potency typical antipsychotics, or high dose.
- Prophylaxis with anticholinergic agent for first month of treatment in those with high risk or previous history.
- May be very frightening and painful for the patient.
- Can occur in a tardive form, with symptoms lasting for greater than 6 months after discontinuation of the offending agent.

Fun Fact:
Dystonia has many causes other than antipsychotics, and is the third most common movement disorder in the United States, following essential tremor and Parkinson's disease. Neurologists use botulinum toxin (Botox) to treat some dystonias, especially cervical dystonias.

Excessive Sweating (Hyperhidrosis)

Characteristics: Excessive sweating, which tends to be more prominent in the face, neck, and chest, and less prominent in the armpits and palms.

Meds That Cause It: Antidepressants, especially SNRIs (venlafaxine, duloxetine, levomilnacipran) and bupropion.

Mechanism: Dysregulation of cholinergically innervated sweat glands.

General Management:

Reduce dose or switch agents.

First-Line Medications:

- Terazosin (alpha-1 blocker); start 1 mg at bedtime, then gradually increase up to 4 mg–6 mg (SE: Dizziness, dry mouth, hypotension, rebound hypertension if stopped abruptly).
- Clonidine 0.1 mg daily.
- Benztropine 1 mg BID.
- Glycopyrrolate; start 1 mg twice daily and increase gradually up to 2 mg 3 times a day. Can be used PRN.

Second-Line Medications:

- Oxybutynin 5 mg–10 mg daily or twice daily.
- Mirtazapine up to 60 mg daily as adjunct.
- Cyproheptadine 4 mg daily or twice daily.
- Aripiprazole 10 mg daily (one trial showed it alleviated hyperhidrosis due to fluoxetine or duloxetine).

Clinical Pearls:

- Patients may not need to take medication for sweating in the winter.
- Often occurs in people who tended to sweat a lot before taking the medication.

Fun Fact:

Glycopyrrolate is so effective at reducing sweating that the label warns it can reduce the body's ability to cool off by sweating—which, in very high temperatures, can cause fever and heatstroke.

Fatigue

Characteristics: Sleepiness as a result of medications, usually due to antidepressants. Typically, patients say they sleep more than enough at night, yet they feel like they could fall asleep at any point throughout the day.

Meds That Cause It: Antidepressants (especially paroxetine, mirtazapine, and tricyclics; bupropion is *least* likely to cause fatigue); antipsychotics (especially clozapine, quetiapine, olanzapine, ziprasidone, but all can cause it); mood stabilizers; benztropine; antihistamines (eg, diphenhydramine); opiates.

Mechanism: Various mechanisms, often due to antihistamine or anticholinergic effects.

General Management:

- Watchful waiting for spontaneous resolution (not usually effective).
- Change dosing to bedtime.
- Reduce dose.

Medications:

- Psychostimulants such as methylphenidate or dexedrine. Depending on the response, you may switch to a long-acting stimulant eventually.
- Modafinil (Provigil) 100–300 mg daily in divided doses.
- Armodafinil (Nuvigil) 150–250 mg daily in divided doses.
- If a serotonergic antidepressant is causing fatigue, consider switching to bupropion.

Clinical Pearls:

- Rule out non-medication causes of fatigue, such as obstructive sleep apnea, hypothyroidism, and anemia.
- Fatigue can be a residual symptom of partially treated depression.
- If patients are taking a benzodiazepine for anxiety or insomnia, this could be causing daytime fatigue. Consider decreasing the dose or switching to a different agent.

Fun Fact:

Some consider the US to be the most overworked developed country. The number of hours Americans work (86% of men and 67% of women work more than 40 hours weekly) and the absence of a national paid parental leave benefit contribute to this distinction, as does the lack of federal laws requiring maximum work week length, paid sick leave, or vacation days. No wonder so many experience fatigue.

Nausea

Characteristics: Nausea or sensation of upset stomach beginning soon after first dose of a new medication.

Meds That Cause It: Serotonergic antidepressants (especially vortioxetine), lithium, valproic acid, naltrexone.

Mechanism: Various; may be related to stimulation of 5-HT-3 receptors.

General Management:

- Reduce dose.
- Wait 1–2 weeks, since nausea is often transient.
- Switch to a non-serotonergic antidepressant.
- Start drug at half the usual dose and go up gradually.
- Take medication just after meals.
- Split the dose into BID or TID dosing.
- Switch to a delayed release, extended release, or enteric coated formulation, if available (eg, valproic acid, lithium).
- Take a spoonful of peanut butter before taking the medication.

Medications (SE: Most well tolerated especially when used PRN; sedation common with many)

- Ginger root capsules 2 caps 2–3 times per day.
- Trimethobenzamide (Tigan) 300 mg TID PRN.
- Promethazine (Phenergan) 12.5 mg–25 mg BID PRN.
- Ondansetron (Zofran) 4 mg–8 mg Q 8 hours PRN (5-HT-3 blocker).
- Mirtazapine (Remeron) 15 mg daily (5-HT-3 blocker).
- Metoclopramide (Reglan) 10 mg 3 times a day as needed.
- Prochlorperazine (Compazine) 5–10 mg Q 8 hours PRN.

Clinical Pearls:

- Both metoclopramide and prochlorperazine are phenothiazines and, like others in that class, may cause EPS if continued for too long.
- Patients with preexisting GERD may be more susceptible to med-induced nausea. Try prescribing a proton pump inhibitor, such as omeprazole (Prilosec), along with the offending agent.

Fun Fact:

Antipsychotics rarely cause nausea—in fact, several are FDA-approved anti-emetics.

Orthostatic Hypotension (Postural Hypotension)

Characteristics: Orthostatic hypotension (OH) is caused by blood pooling in the lower extremities when people stand up, causing less blood flow to the brain and consequent dizziness. Usually caused by medications that block the alpha-1 receptors, which are responsible for telling the body to constrict blood vessels (and maintain blood pressure) after standing up. Patients will report feeling faint when they get up, and occasionally a sense of the room spinning (vertigo).

Meds That Cause It: Antipsychotics, especially clozapine, risperidone, quetiapine, and lower-potency typical agents. Antidepressants, especially tricyclics, MAOIs, trazodone, sometimes mirtazapine.

Mechanism: Alpha-1 receptor blockade, also anticholinergic effects.

General Management:

- Review all meds, including non-psychiatric, since many blood pressure and cardiac meds, as well as alpha blockers like prazosin (Minipress) and tamsulosin (Flomax) used for benign prostatic hyperplasia, can cause OH.
- Start at lower dose and titrate more slowly, especially when using higher-risk agents in higher-risk patients.
- Change dosing to minimize peak blood levels (eg, split dosing or switch to an extended release version).
- Instruct patient to stand up slowly.
- Prevent dehydration by drinking enough fluids.
- Compression stockings, also known as TED stockings.
- Increase salt intake (if no hypertension).
- Limit alcohol use.

Medications:

- Fludrocortisone (Florinef) 0.1 mg daily; can increase to 0.3 mg daily. SE: Hypokalemia. Use only in severe cases where other measures have not worked.
- Midodrine 10 mg 3 times daily. SE: Goose bumps, paresthesias. Use only in severe cases where other measures have not worked.

Clinical Pearls:

- Orthostatic hypotension is defined as a 20 mm drop in systolic pressure or a 10 mm drop in diastolic pressure within 3 minutes of a patient moving from lying to standing position.
- Ask patients when the symptom is worse; if it is worse an hour or two after taking the medication, it is most likely medication-induced.
- More common and problematic in elderly; may contribute to fall risk.

Fun Fact:

A recent epidemiologic observational study out of Johns Hopkins, following nearly 12,000 individuals over 20 years, recently suggested that OH in middle age increases risk of cognitive decline and later dementia.

Parkinsonism

Characteristics: Also known as pseudoparkinsonism, these drug-induced symptoms mimic the symptoms of Parkinson's disease:

- Tremor (especially apparent in the hands as a "pill rolling" tremor).
- Rigidity (cog-wheel rigidity).
- Bradykinesia (slow movement), decreased arm swing.
- Shuffling gait.
- Slurred speech.
- Mask-like facies, stooped posture, drooling.
- Psychological side effects, such as cognitive dulling (bradyphrenia), worse negative symptoms (neuroleptic-induced deficit syndrome), worse depression (neuroleptic dysphoria).

Meds That Cause It: Antipsychotics, especially typical agents, but atypical antipsychotics may also cause it. Least likely to cause it are clozapine, olanzapine, quetiapine, and ziprasidone.

Mechanism: D2 blockade, disruption of the balance between dopaminergic vs cholinergic neurons.

General Management:

Decrease dose or switch to a different antipsychotic.

First-Line Medications:

- Benztropine 1 mg–2 mg once or twice per day.
- Trihexyphenidyl 2 mg–5 mg once or twice per day.
- Diphenhydramine 50 mg/day.

Second-Line Medications:

Amantadine 100 mg–200 mg twice per day (enhances dopamine release).

Clinical Pearls:

- May occur at any time, but typically seen within 1–2 months after antipsychotic is initiated.
- Highest-risk patients: Female, older, higher-potency agents, higher doses.
- In patients at high risk of parkinsonism, start benztropine (or one of the other first-line agents) at the same time as starting the antipsychotic.
- Try discontinuing the anticholinergic agent after several weeks; many patients will not need to remain on it long term.

Fun Fact:

Parkinson's disease is named after Dr. James Parkinson (1755–1824), the doctor who first identified the condition. It's caused by loss of neurons in the substantia nigra, where most dopamine is produced.

QT Interval Prolongation

Characteristics: The QT interval in the cardiac cycle represents depolarization (contraction) and repolarization (relaxation) of ventricles (these interval times are corrected to account for variations in heart rate, specified as "QTc"). Normal QTc intervals are generally defined as <460 msec for women and <450 msec for men. QT prolongation can lead to serious arrhythmias, including torsades de pointes (TdP), and sudden death. While the link between QT and TdP is not clear, QTc above 500 msec is a significant risk factor for TdP.

Meds That Cause It: Typical antipsychotics (especially thioridazine, high doses of chlorpromazine, and intravenous haloperidol). Of atypical antipsychotics, ziprasidone has greatest risk of prolonging QT, though to a lower degree. Of SSRIs, higher-dose citalopram (>40 mg/day) most likely. Of TCAs, amitriptyline and maprotiline. Methadone. In overdose, a large number of medications can prolong QT.

Mechanism: The mechanism depends on the offending drug. For example, TCAs prolong the QT through blockade of sodium and calcium channels, while citalopram and chlorpromazine do so through blockade of potassium channels.

Management:

- Prevent: Identify risk factors (see below), get baseline electrolytes, ECG, and monitor periodically in patients at risk.
- With prolonged QTc (>500 msec), obtain a cardiologist consult.
- In patients with a borderline QTc, switch to a less risky agent.
  - Lower-risk antipsychotics: Aripiprazole has minimal risk; asenapine, lurasidone, olanzapine, and quetiapine are also good options.
  - Lower-risk antidepressants: All antidepressants at usual therapeutic doses are relatively safe (avoid citalopram >40 mg/day). However, sertraline may be the best choice because it is the most studied in cardiac patients and has few drug interactions.

Clinical Pearls:

- Risk factors: Congenital (long QT syndrome), female gender, older age, electrolyte abnormalities (low potassium, calcium, magnesium), and other conditions such as hepatic dysfunction, diabetes, hypothyroidism, AIDS, and hypertension.
- Heart conditions that increase a patient's risk are bradycardia, left ventricular dysfunction, heart failure, mitral valve prolapse, and myocardial infarction.
- Caution in situations that may affect electrolytes, including eating disorders, diuretic use, hypoglycemia, renal dysfunction, and pituitary insufficiency.
- Other common medications that are not related to psychiatry can also be culprits, including antiarrhythmics such as sotalol, amiodarone, and quinidine; macrolide antibiotics such as azithromycin; quinolone antibiotics such as levofloxacin; some antifungals; antimalarials; and other medications such as tamoxifen.
- Overdose with psychotropic medication, even "low risk" agents, can lead to QT prolongation.

Fun Fact:

- *Torsades de pointes* translates to "twisting of the points," illustrating the chaotic nature of the heart rhythm that can lead to sudden death.

Sexual Dysfunction

Characteristics: Impairment of some aspect of sexual functioning, including low libido, anorgasmia, decreased sensation, erectile dysfunction, or delayed or retrograde ejaculation (in men).

Meds That Cause It: Antidepressants (paroxetine most likely, but all SSRIs and SNRIs can cause it); antipsychotics (primarily risperidone and paliperidone); some mood stabilizers (valproic acid and carbamazepine).

Mechanism: Various, including activation of 5-HT-2 receptors by antidepressants; hyperprolactinemia by antipsychotics such as risperidone; and anticholinergic and antiadrenergic effects in other antipsychotics, especially first generation.

General Management:

- Watchful waiting—works in 10%–20% of patients.
- Drug holiday—no dose Friday or Saturday, resume Sunday or Monday. (Not a good idea with paroxetine or venlafaxine due to discontinuation syndrome, nor with fluoxetine due to long half-life.)
- Decrease dose.
- Switch to a medication with low sexual side effects (eg, bupropion, mirtazapine, or an antipsychotic that does not affect prolactin).

First-Line Medications:

- Add a PDE-5 inhibitor, such as sildenafil (Viagra) or tadalafil (Cialis). Works best for erectile dysfunction, but may help with low libido as well. Less effective in women.
- Add bupropion (possibly more effective in women than men).

Second-Line Medications:

- Buspirone 30 mg–60 mg daily.
- Periactin 8 mg 30 minutes before sex.
- Amantadine 100 mg daily.

Clinical Pearls:

It can be hard to know if sexual dysfunction (SD) is caused by a medication, the underlying psychiatric condition, or a separate problem predating the medication. For this reason, you should try to obtain a sexual history in your patients before starting medications that can cause SD.

Fun Fact:

Early estimates of SD incidence from antidepressants were very low (in the range of 2%–16%) because researchers relied on spontaneous self-reporting. By contrast, in a prospective study of 1,022 outpatients, all of whom were asked specifically about sexual functioning, the authors estimated that SSRIs and venlafaxine caused rates of SD ranging from 58% to 73% (Montejo AL, *J Clin Psych* 2001;62 Suppl 3:10–21).

Sialorrhea (Hypersalivation)

Characteristics: Excessive drooling, usually more severe at night.

Meds That Cause It: Clozapine is the most common cause (30%–80% incidence). Can be caused by olanzapine, risperidone, or quetiapine.

Mechanism: Pro-cholinergic effect.

General Management:

- Chew sugarless gum, which encourages more frequent swallowing of saliva.
- Place towel over pillow if main bothersome symptom is nocturnal sialorrhea.

First-Line Medications:

Glycopyrrolate (Robinul): Start 1 mg at bedtime, then increase to 1 mg–2 mg twice daily if symptoms are prominent during the day. Unlike other anticholinergics, glycopyrrolate does not cross the blood-brain barrier, so there are fewer central anticholinergic side effects. SE: Constipation, dry mouth, blurred vision, urinary retention.

Second-Line Medications:

- Ipratropium (Atrovent) 0.03% nasal spray; use 1–2 sprays sublingually (rather than intranasally).
- Oxybutinin (Ditropan) 5 mg twice daily.
- Alpha agonists such as clonidine (0.05 mg–0.1 mg daily or weekly transdermal patch 0.1 mg–0.2 mg) or guanfacine.
- Benztropine (Cogentin) 1 mg twice daily.
- Trihexyphenidyl (Artane) 5 mg twice daily.
- Atropine 1% ophthalmic drops; use 1 drop TID PRN sublingually.

Clinical Pearls:

- Dose reduction of clozapine usually is not helpful in diminishing symptoms.
- Clozapine has strong anticholinergic properties, so its pro-cholinergic effect of excessive drooling is puzzling. Theories explaining this include specific stimulation of cholinergic salivary receptors and impairment in the autonomically mediated swallowing mechanism (which may also contribute to clozapine-related dysphagia and pneumonia).

Fun Fact:

Ayurvedic medicine recommends a number of natural treatments for hypersalivation, including chewing cloves, drinking cinnamon tea, and eating a combination of pepper, ginger, and honey.

Tardive Dyskinesia

Characteristics: Involuntary movements, usually occurring after months or years of antipsychotic treatment. The most common symptoms are oro-buccal-lingual, such as chewing, lip smacking, and tongue protrusion. Occasionally causes movements of fingers or toes.

Meds That Cause It: Antipsychotics, especially first-generation antipsychotics (3%–5% per year); the risk is smaller with second-generation antipsychotics. Among SGAs, risperidone confers the highest risk.

Mechanism: D2 blockade leading to dopamine receptor supersensitivity.

General Management:

- Monitor all patients taking antipsychotics regularly with a test such as the AIMS (Abnormal Involuntary Movement Scale).
- Switch to a different antipsychotic, preferably a low-potency SGA, such as olanzapine, quetiapine, or clozapine.

First-Line Medications:

- Valbenazine (Ingrezza) 40 mg/day; increase to 80 mg/day after a week. SE: Sedation, akathisia. FDA approved for TD.
- Deutetrabenazine (Austedo): Start 6 mg once BID; increase weekly by 6 mg/day increments to maximum dose of 48 mg/day (divide doses >12 mg/day BID).
- Tetrabenazine (Xenazine): Start 12.5 mg QD for one week, increase by 12.5 mg/day increments weekly to usual dose of 75 mg–150 mg QD (divided doses >37.5 mg TID). SE: Sedation, akathisia, tremor. FDA approved for Huntington's disease.

Second-Line Medications:

- Amantadine 100 mg–300 mg/day.
- Gingko biloba extract 240 mg/day.
- Vitamin E 400 IU–600 IU/day.
- Benzodiazepines (eg, clonazepam or lorazepam 0.5–1 mg daily or BID).

Clinical Pearls:

- Risk factors for TD include FGAs as opposed to SGAs, higher-potency agents, duration of exposure, higher dose, elderly, African American.
- Increasing the dose of the antipsychotic will improve symptoms temporarily but probably make them worse in the long run.
- Decreasing or discontinuing antipsychotics may often worsen the symptoms temporarily ("withdrawal dyskinesia") or even unmask TD symptoms that were not apparent.

Fun Fact:

Antipsychotics aren't the only medications that may cause TD. Prolonged use of medications for nausea and reflux like metoclopramide (Reglan) and prochlorperazine (Compazine), which also block dopamine, have also been associated with TD.

Tremor

Characteristics: Rapid regular movements of body parts, especially hands. Classified as fine vs coarse, and as resting vs postural vs intention.

Meds That Cause It: Lithium (fine intention tremor), valproic acid (fine), lamotrigine, bupropion, antipsychotics (Parkinsonian, resting coarse tremor), especially high-potency typical agents, risperidone. Occasionally SSRIs and buspirone.

Mechanism: Multiple mechanisms depending on cause. Medication-induced tremor may be induced by excitability in muscle receptors and neuronal reflexes.

General Management:

- Rule out unrelated causes, such as essential tremor or hyperthyroidism.
- Most drug tremors are fine postural tremor (seen best when patient is holding a fixed posture, such as holding hands up with arms extended).
- Reduce use of caffeine, which can worsen all tremors.
- Change dosing to minimize peak blood levels (eg, split dosing, switch to an extended release version, or give full dose before sleep).
- Reduce dose or switch agents.

First-Line Medications:

- Propranolol 10 mg BID as needed, can go up to 30 mg–120 mg daily in 2 or 3 divided doses. SE: Dizziness, fatigue, syncope, low BP.
- Inderal LA. Long-acting propranolol that can be dosed 60 mg–80 mg once a day.
- Benztropine 1 mg BID for Parkinsonian tremor (due to antipsychotics).

Second-Line Medications:

- Primidone 100 mg 3 times a day.
- Vitamin B6 for lithium tremor 900 mg–1200 mg daily.
- Amantadine 100 mg–200 mg BID for Parkinsonian tremor (due to antipsychotics).
- Various anticonvulsants such as topiramate, gabapentin, oxcarbazepine.

Clinical Pearls:

- Try to systematically track the severity of the tremor over time. Options include taking a quick video at each appointment, having patients copy a design or write their name and address, or having them drink a cup of water. Take notes or include samples during visits.
- Don't forget that tremor can signal alcohol or benzodiazepine withdrawal—something you might want to ask patients about.

Fun Fact:

One in 5 people over the age of 65 may have essential tremor (not associated with medication).

Weight Gain

Characteristics: Typically, patients will report food craving and binging. Weight gain rapid in first 3 months, more gradual over following year, then often plateaus. Rapid initial weight gain is correlated with greater eventual cumulative weight gain. FDA definition of weight gain is ≥7% increase in weight from baseline.

Meds That Cause It: Antipsychotics, especially clozapine, olanzapine, and quetiapine. Somewhat less weight gain with risperidone and paliperidone. Least weight gain with aripiprazole, haloperidol, ziprasidone, and lurasidone. Antidepressants: Mirtazapine, tricyclics, paroxetine. Mood stabilizers: Lithium, valproic acid.

Mechanism: Blockade of histamine and serotonin 2A receptors, leading to increased hunger.

General Management:

- Monitoring: Weight, BMI, waist circumference every 4 weeks for 3 months, then every 3 months.
- Lifestyle modification, including exercise and dietary changes, is helpful for patients who are motivated; several studies have shown some benefit, but in actual clinical settings it may be difficult to match their results.
- Switch to a medication that is more weight neutral.

First-Line Medications: (some evidence specifically for reducing psychotropic-induced weight gain)

- Topiramate 100 mg–300 mg/day; SE: Cognitive dulling.
- Metformin XR 500 mg–2000 mg: Take with largest meal, split into 2 doses if needed (based on GI side effects).
- Orlistat 120 mg 3 times daily after meals. Interferes with fat absorption; SE: Diarrhea.
- Aripiprazole 15 mg/day. Antipsychotic. May be useful for olanzapine-induced weight gain as adjunct.

Second-Line Medications: (effective for weight loss, but little or no evidence specifically for psychotropic-induced weight gain)

- Bupropion SR 300 mg–400 mg daily.
- Any psychostimulant either methylphenidate or amphetamine class.
- Naltrexone/bupropion (Contrave) 8 mg/90 mg up to 2 tabs twice daily. Anti-obesity drug.
- Phentermine (Suprenza) 15 mg–37.5 mg daily. Anti-obesity drug.
- Phentermine/topiramate (Qsymia) 7.5 mg/46 mg up to 2 tabs daily. Anti-obesity drug.
- Zonisamide (Zonegran) 100 mg–600 mg/day. Anticonvulsant.
- Nizatidine (Axid) 150 mg–300 mg daily. Antacid, H-2 blocker, available OTC.
- Amantadine (Symmetrel) 100 mg–300 mg/day.

Clinical Pearls:

- Weight gain is most likely in the first 6 weeks of taking an antipsychotic, and it's difficult for patients to ever lose this weight. As such, you should monitor weekly initially, and switch to a more weight-neutral agent at the first sign of weight gain.
- If patient gains 5% or more of body weight, switch to a different drug.
- Ziprasidone and aripiprazole are probably the most weight-neutral antipsychotics and may even cause weight loss, especially if switching from another agent.
- Weight gain tends to be most severe in patients who are taking an antipsychotic for the first time.
- Ask weight-gaining patients about dry mouth; many psychotropics cause this, and such patients may gain weight from drinking sugary beverages to deal with this side effect.

Fun Fact:

Some researchers have hypothesized that treatment-emergent weight gain is related to and predictive of clinical response, but others argue it may be a marker for medication adherence instead.

Sleep Disorder Medications

GENERAL PRESCRIBING TIPS

There are only 4 medications in this section—modafinil (Provigil), armodafinil (Nuvigil), sodium oxybate (Xyrem), and tasimelteon (Hetlioz). In reality, very few of you will ever prescribe Xyrem or Hetlioz. Xyrem is approved for narcolepsy with cataplexy, which is a rare illness treated by sleep specialists, and Hetlioz is used for another rare condition seen primarily in the blind, non-24-hour sleep-wake disorder (N24SWD).

The two "vigil" drugs, on the other hand, are pretty heavily prescribed by psychiatrists for all manner of situations. Some are legitimate (shift-work disorder, jet lag, antidepressant-induced sleepiness), and others, undisclosed to the prescribers, are pretty marginal (staying up all night to study—or to party). These meds, along with the stimulants, are often used as "cognitive enhancers" by over-achievers. Whether that's a good or a bad thing is a subject of ongoing debate.

These "wake promoting" agents are often prescribed when patients complain of excessive fatigue. In these clinical scenarios, we recommend a thorough workup to determine potential other strategies (eg, labs to rule out hypothyroidism, anemia, and other conditions; a sleep study to rule out apnea or restless leg syndrome; a review of medications or other substances potentially contributing to daytime sedation; and education on good sleep habits).

There's no clear guidance on which of the vigils to prescribe. Nuvigil lasts a few hours longer than Provigil, which can be a blessing for those who want to stay awake longer or a curse for those who find it causes them insomnia. Trial and error is the way to go with these agents.

TABLE 15: Sleep Disorder Medications

Generic Name (Brand Name) Year FDA Approved *[G] denotes generic availability*	Relevant FDA Indication(s)	Rx Status	Available Strengths	Usual Dosage Range (starting–max)
Armodafinil [G] (Nuvigil) 2007	Excessive sleepiness (OSA, narcolepsy, shift-work)	Schedule IV	50, 150, 200, 250 mg	150–250 mg/day
Modafinil [G] (Provigil) 1998	Excessive sleepiness (OSA, narcolepsy, shift-work)	Schedule IV	100, 200 mg	100–400 mg/day
Sodium oxybate (Xyrem) 2002	Cataplexy and excessive daytime sedation (narcolepsy)	Schedule III	0.5 g/mL	6–9 g/night
Tasimelteon (Hetlioz) 2014	Non-24-hour sleep-wake disorder	Rx	20	20 mg/night

ARMODAFINIL (Nuvigil) Fact Sheet [G]

FDA Indications:
Excessive sleepiness associated with obstructive sleep apnea, narcolepsy, or shift-work disorder.

Off-Label Uses:
ADHD; fatigue; treatment-resistant depression.

Dosage Forms:
Tablets: 50 mg, 150 mg, 200 mg, 250 mg.

Dosage Guidance:
- Obstructive sleep apnea or narcolepsy: 150 mg–250 mg QAM.
- Shift-work sleep disorder: 150 mg QD, 1 hour before start of work shift.

Monitoring: No routine monitoring recommended unless clinical picture warrants.

Cost: $$

Side Effects:
- Most common: Headache, nausea, dizziness, insomnia, anxiety, irritability.
- Serious but rare: Serious rash, including Stevens-Johnson syndrome, multi-organ hypersensitivity reaction, angioedema, and anaphylaxis reported rarely. Rare cases of mania, psychosis, and agitation reported.

Mechanism, Pharmacokinetics, and Drug Interactions:
- Dopamine reuptake inhibitor.
- Metabolized primarily by non-CYP450 liver pathways, but also to some degree by CYP3A4; t ½: 15 hours.
- Duration of action about 8 hours.
- Potentially induces CYP1A2 and 3A4 and inhibits 2C19. Avoid concomitant use with steroidal contraceptives (hormone levels may be decreased due to 3A4 induction) and with CYP2C19 substrates (eg, omeprazole, phenytoin, diazepam); levels of these medications may be increased.

Clinical Pearls:
- Armodafinil is, as the name implies, the R-modafinil enantiomer (modafinil is a 1:1 mixture of both R- and S-enantiomers).
- Schedule IV controlled substance due to abuse potential, mostly for euphoric and stimulant-like effects.
- Increased heart rate and blood pressure may occur, particularly in patients who don't suffer from excessive sedation or fatigue and when used at higher doses.

Fun Fact:
In 2010, the FDA declined to approve use of Nuvigil to treat jet lag.

Bottom Line:
Effective wake-promoting agent with some potential for abuse and for drug interactions. Lasts a bit longer than modafinil.

MODAFINIL (Provigil) Fact Sheet [G]

FDA Indications:
Excessive sleepiness associated with obstructive sleep apnea, narcolepsy, or shift-work disorder.

Off-Label Uses:
ADHD; fatigue; treatment-resistant depression.

Dosage Forms:
Tablets (G): 100 mg, 200 mg.

Dosage Guidance:
- Obstructive sleep apnea or narcolepsy: 100 mg–400 mg QAM (usually 200 mg QAM).
- Shift-work sleep disorder: 100 mg–400 mg QD (usually 200 mg QAM), 1 hour before start of work shift.
- ADHD (off-label): 100 mg–400 mg QAM.
- Treatment-resistant depression, bipolar or unipolar (off-label): 100 mg–400 mg QAM added to antidepressant.

Monitoring: No routine monitoring recommended unless clinical picture warrants.

Cost: $$

Side Effects:
- Most common: Increased heart rate and blood pressure, headache, nausea, jitteriness, rhinitis, diarrhea, back pain, and insomnia.
- Serious but rare: Serious rash, including Stevens-Johnson syndrome, multi-organ hypersensitivity reaction, angioedema, and anaphylaxis reported rarely. Rare cases of mania, psychosis, and agitation reported.

Mechanism, Pharmacokinetics, and Drug Interactions:
- Dopamine reuptake inhibitor.
- Metabolized primarily by non-CYP450 liver pathways, but also to some degree by CYP3A4; t ½: 15 hours.
- Duration of action about 6 hours.
- Potentially induces CYP1A2 and 3A4 and inhibits 2C19. Avoid concomitant use with steroidal contraceptives (hormone levels may be decreased due to 3A4 induction) and with CYP2C9/19 substrates (eg, omeprazole, phenytoin, diazepam); levels of these medications may be increased.

Clinical Pearls:
- Schedule IV controlled substance.
- Increased heart rate and blood pressure may occur, particularly in patients who don't suffer from excessive sedation or fatigue and at higher doses.

Fun Fact:
An ADHD indication was rejected by the FDA because of modafinil's possible association with Stevens-Johnson syndrome.

Bottom Line:
While modafinil can be helpful for many causes of excessive sleepiness, realize that many people end up using it off-label for lifestyle enhancement, such as working, studying, and partying longer.

SODIUM OXYBATE (Xyrem) Fact Sheet

FDA Indications:
Cataplexy and excessive daytime sedation in narcolepsy.

Off-Label Uses:
Fibromyalgia; chronic pain; neuropathic pain.

Dosage Forms:
Oral solution: 0.5 g/mL.

Dosage Guidance:
Start 4.5 g nightly, given in 2 equal, divided doses (because of extremely short half-life): 2.25 g at bedtime and 2.25 g taken 2.5–4 hours later. Titrate to effect in increments of 1.5 g/night at weekly intervals (0.75 g at bedtime and 0.75 g taken 2.5–4 hours later). Usual dose 6 g–9 g per night. Max 9 g/night.

Monitoring: No routine monitoring recommended unless clinical picture warrants.

Cost: $$$$$

Side Effects:
- Most common: Nausea, dizziness, vomiting, somnolence, enuresis, tremor, parasomnias (sleepwalking).
- Serious but rare: Respiratory depression, depression and suicidality, impaired motor and cognitive function.

Mechanism, Pharmacokinetics, and Drug Interactions:
- CNS depressant.
- Metabolized primarily by conversion to carbon dioxide and then eliminated by expiration; t ½: 0.5–1 hour.
- Avoid concomitant use with alcohol, sedative hypnotics, and other CNS depressants. Valproic acid increases sodium oxybate levels by 25%; adjust valproic acid dose by at least 20%.

Clinical Pearls:
- Sodium oxybate is the sodium salt of gamma hydroxybutyrate (GHB), a Schedule I controlled substance ("date rape" drug).
- Sodium oxybate is a Schedule III controlled substance and is available only through a restricted distribution program called the Xyrem REMS Program using a centralized pharmacy. Prescribers and patients must enroll in the program (https://www.xyremrems.com or 1-866-XYREM88).
- Patient must wait at least 2 hours after eating before taking a dose. Both doses should be prepared (dilute in provided vials with water) before bedtime. Dose must be taken while in bed, and patient is to lie down after dosing.
- Most patients find the taste of Xyrem to be awful.
- Xyrem alone was just as effective as modafinil alone for excessive daytime sedation, but the combination was significantly better than either medication used alone in one narcolepsy study.

Fun Fact:
Xyrem, an orphan drug, is expensive, between $108,000 and $160,000 per year depending on the nightly dose. Jazz Pharmaceuticals is looking to expand its use by testing it in obstructive sleep apnea, Parkinson's, chronic fatigue, schizophrenia, binge eating, and cluster headache.

Bottom Line:
Xyrem is often used by sleep specialists as a first-line agent for narcolepsy with cataplexy. It's unlikely that many psychiatrists will ever prescribe it, given its dangers.

TASIMELTEON (Hetlioz) Fact Sheet

FDA Indications:
Non-24-hour sleep-wake disorder (N24SWD).

Off-Label Uses:
None recommended; potentially may be used for insomnia, jet lag, shift-work disorder.

Dosage Forms:
Capsules: 20 mg.

Dosage Guidance:
Start 20 mg QHS at the same time every night.

Monitoring: No routine monitoring recommended unless clinical picture warrants.

Cost: $$$$$

Side Effects:
- Most common: Headache, increased LFTs, nightmares or unusual dreams.
- Serious but rare: None reported.

Mechanism, Pharmacokinetics, and Drug Interactions:
- Melatonin receptor agonist (at both MT1 and MT2 receptors).
- Metabolized primarily by CYP1A2 and 3A4; t ½: 1 hour.
- Smoking may reduce tasimelteon levels by 40% and lower its efficacy. Caution with 3A4 inhibitors and inducers.

Clinical Pearls:
- Like ramelteon, tasimelteon binds melatonin receptors. Tasimelteon has greater affinity for the MT2 receptor, whereas ramelteon has greater affinity for the MT1 receptor. Both are fairly non-selective, though (meaning they both bind to both MT1 and MT2), so making a clinical distinction is difficult.
- Approved as an orphan drug (a drug for rare diseases that affect fewer than 200,000 people).
- N24SWD is a circadian rhythm disorder commonly seen in blind patients with no light perception. Due to absence of environmental input, these patients experience a constant gradual shift of their sleep cycles by roughly 30 minutes per day, re-aligning with the 24-hour clock only once every 48 days.
- Should be used daily to maintain therapeutic effect.

Fun Fact:
The advocacy group Public Citizen accused the FDA of allowing tasimelteon's manufacturer to list N24SWD as the drug's indication without specifying that it was for use in totally blind people with N24SWD, the originally filed indication for consideration. Rather than correcting the error and adjusting the drug's label, the FDA sent out a press release officially expanding the approved indication to any patients with N24SWD (there are sighted individuals with this disorder, likely with a genetic basis).

Bottom Line:
At over $13,000 for a month's supply, this drug should be used only in patients with N24SWD. Even in this case, though, you may want to consider ramelteon. While ramelteon hasn't been studied in patients with N24SWD, it's reasonable to try because it is so similar pharmacologically yet much more affordable.

Substance Abuse/ Dependence Medications

GENERAL PRESCRIBING TIPS

Although medications are helpful in substance abuse, you should combine them with other approaches, such as therapy and 12-step programs. Most patients with substance abuse issues have co-occurring psychiatric disorders. Some clinicians prefer to get the substance abuse under control before treating other disorders, under the theory that substances can both obscure and aggravate the underlying psychiatric symptoms. In practice, however, it takes patients a very long time to get sober, and treatment of other conditions usually can't wait. For more detailed practical guidance on treating addiction, check out *Addiction Treatment: A Carlat Guide* by Michael Weaver, MD.

Opioid Dependence

- Methadone was first approved by the FDA for use in opioid dependence in 1947. It is a substitute therapy, and while it rarely gets patients off of opiates, it does help decrease the use of illicit forms of opiates. The problem is that patients must show up at methadone clinics to receive their dose (though they can often eventually qualify for take-home doses), making it hard to carve out a normal work or family life.
- Buprenorphine/naloxone combination (Suboxone and others) was approved in 2002 and has many advantages over methadone. You can give patients a 30-day supply, allowing them to avoid the methadone lifestyle. Buprenorphine/naloxone is probably also a little easier to taper off of than methadone for patients who want to attain total opiate sobriety.

Alcohol Dependence

- Disulfiram (Antabuse) is an aversive treatment, causing patients to become ill if they drink while taking the medication. For a long time it was the only approved medication for treating alcohol dependence, and it still has a place in treatment for patients who are very highly motivated to not drink at all (for example, those who are on probation after a DUI, or those who are about to lose jobs or partners if they go on just one more bender).
- Naltrexone (ReVia, Vivitrol) blocks a specific type of opiate receptor in the brain, and is thought to act by reducing cravings and the rewarding effects of alcohol. Most substance abuse specialists consider it the treatment of choice for alcoholism.
- Acamprosate (Campral) is effective in maintaining abstinence after detox. It is thought to "normalize" the brain glutamate system, which becomes unstable after many years of heavy alcohol use. It may work best in patients who are not abusing other substances, who are alcohol-free before starting it, and who have a strong commitment to abstinence.
- Combining medications is another strategy. For example, the combination of acamprosate and disulfiram seems to be more effective than acamprosate alone; however, the combination of naltrexone and acamprosate has not been shown to be more effective than naltrexone alone.

Smoking Cessation

See our special smoking cessation fact sheet in this section for more information.

Smoking Cessation

(The following is adapted from a Carlat One-Pager that was originally created for the June 2015 issue of the *Carlat Addiction Treatment Report*. See that issue for the full article.)

Assessment

DSM-5: "Problematic pattern" of tobacco use leading to "significant distress" that lasts at least 12 months.

1. *Determine daily nicotine use.* How many packs per day (20 mg nicotine is typically absorbed per 20-cigarette pack)? E-cigarettes (nicotine varies)? Chewing tobacco (1 pouch = ¼ pack)? Hookah?
2. *Determine the usage pattern.* When does the patient have the day's first cigarette? Does the patient smoke when sick?
3. *Determine past quitting techniques.* Have any worked—or *not* worked?

Pharmacological Treatment: Which to Choose?

- **Nicotine replacement therapy (NRT).** Start most patients on NRT. Prescribe patch based on nicotine load: 1 ppd = 21 mg patch. Place it at the same time each day, usually in the morning. Start above the heart and rotate left around the body to prevent skin irritation. Use 0.5% cortisone cream for irritation/rash. Initial dose for 4–8 weeks, then taper monthly or every 2 months. Advise no smoking—patients may note nausea or racing heart if they do.
- **Combination NRT.** If there are cravings throughout the day even with a patch, add a short-acting agent (gum, lozenge, spray, inhaler). Discuss chewing technique for gum: Chew a few times to activate the release (the sign is bad peppery taste), then park between cheek and gum, and switch sides every few minutes. Each piece is 2 mg or 4 mg and lasts about 30 minutes. Spray and inhaler are available by prescription only.
- **Varenicline (Chantix).** Start 0.5 mg per day for 3 days, increase to twice daily for 7–10 days, then quit smoking, then increase gradually to 1 mg twice daily for 3 months. Discuss possible insomnia and vivid dreams (common). Psychiatric side effects, such as depression, suicidal ideation, and aggression, are unusual and likely caused by nicotine withdrawal rather than Chantix.
- **Bupropion (Wellbutrin SR, Zyban).** 150 mg/day is just as effective as the manufacturer's recommended dose of 150 mg BID and carries fewer side effects. Possible side effects of insomnia, nervousness, weight loss (potentially good, especially since many people gain weight after quitting).
- Combination NRT is as effective as Chantix. Bupropion is effective, but less so.

Tips to Improve Success of Treatment

- Normalize failure. Most people need multiple quit attempts before success; if patients know this in advance, they might be more willing to come back and try again.
- The first week after quitting is the hardest in terms of craving. Craving spells last 10–20 minutes; distraction techniques can work to deal with them. Patients can try drinking a large glass of cold water, playing a video game, etc.
- Warn patients that they might cough temporarily after they quit—this is a normal lung response to healing.
- Give phone number 1-800-QUIT-NOW for free support.

TABLE 16: Substance Abuse/Dependence Medications

Generic Name (Brand Name) Year FDA Approved (Rx status) *[G] denotes generic availability*	Relevant FDA Indication(s)	Available Strengths (mg)	Usual Dosage Range (mg)
Acamprosate [G] (Campral) 2004 (Rx)	Alcohol	333	666 TID
Buprenorphine [G] (Buprenex, Butrans) 2002 (Schedule III)	Opiate	2, 8 SL 0.3 mg/mL inj (used for pain) 5, 7.5, 10, 15, 20 mcg/h patch (used for pain)	8 QD–16 QD
Buprenorphine extended release injection (Sublocade) 2017 (Schedule III)	Opiate	100, 300	300 mg monthly x2 doses, then 100 mg monthly
Buprenorphine subdermal implant (Probuphine) 2016 (Schedule III)	Opiate	Each implant contains equivalent of 80 mg of buprenorphine	4 implants x1, delivering dose up to 6 months
Buprenorphine and naloxone [G] (Bunavail, Suboxone, Zubsolv) 2002 (Schedule III) Generic available for 2/0.5, 8/2 mg SL tablets only	Opiate	2.1/0.3, 4.2/0.7, 6.3/1 buccal film (Bunavail) 2/0.5, 4/1, 8/2, 12/3 SL film strips (Suboxone) 2/0.5, 8/2 SL tabs (generic only) 1.4/0.36, 2.9/0.71, 5.7/1.4, 8.6/2.1, 11.4/2.9 SL tabs (Zubsolv)	4–24 QD
Bupropion SR [G] (Zyban) 1997 (Rx)	Smoking	150	150 QAM–150 BID
Disulfiram [G] (Antabuse) 1951 (Rx)	Alcohol	250, 500	125 QPM–500 QPM
Methadone [G] (Dolophine, Methadose) 1947 (Schedule II)	Opiate	5, 10, 40 10 mg/mL, 10 mg/5 mL, 5 mg/5 mL oral liquid	20 QD–120 QD
Naloxone (Evzio, Narcan Nasal Spray) 2014 (auto-injector) 2015 (intranasal) (Rx)	Emergency opioid overdose rescue	2 mg/0.4 mL autoinjector 4 mg/0.1 mL intranasal	x1; may repeat every 2–3 minutes
Naltrexone [G] (ReVia) 1984 (Rx)	Alcohol, opiate	50	25 QD–50 QD
Naltrexone ER (Vivitrol) 2006 (Rx)	Alcohol, opiate	380	380 Q 4wk
Nicotine inhaled (Nicotrol Inhaler) 1997 (Rx)	Smoking	4 mg delivered/cartridge	6–16 cartridges per day

Generic Name (Brand Name) Year FDA Approved (Rx status) *[G] denotes generic availability*	Relevant FDA Indication(s)	Available Strengths (mg)	Usual Dosage Range (mg)
Nicotine nasal spray (Nicotrol NS) 1996 (Rx)	Smoking	0.5 mg delivered/spray	1–2 sprays/hour PRN
Nicotine polacrilex [G] (Nicorette Gum, others) 1992 (OTC)	Smoking	2, 4	1 piece PRN up to 24/day
Nicotine polacrilex [G] (Nicorette Lozenge, others) 2009 (OTC)	Smoking	2, 4	1 piece PRN up to 20/day
Nicotine transdermal [G] (Habitrol, Nicoderm CQ) 1991 (OTC)	Smoking	7, 14, 21/24 hours	14–21 QD
Varenicline (Chantix) 2006 (Rx)	Smoking	0.5, 1	0.5 QD–1 BID

ACAMPROSATE (Campral) Fact Sheet [G]

FDA Indications:
Alcohol dependence.

Dosage Forms:
Delayed release tablets (G): 333 mg.

Dosage Guidance:
Start 666 mg TID. Give 333 mg TID in patients with renal impairment.

Monitoring: No routine monitoring recommended unless clinical picture warrants.

Cost: $$$

Side Effects:
- Most common: Diarrhea (dose related, transient), weakness, peripheral edema, insomnia, anxiety.
- Serious but rare: Acute renal failure reported in a few cases; suicidal ideation, attempts, and completions rare but greater than with placebo in studies.

Mechanism, Pharmacokinetics, and Drug Interactions:
- Mechanism of action is not fully defined; it appears to work by promoting a balance between the excitatory and inhibitory neurotransmitters, glutamate and GABA, respectively (GABA and glutamate activities appear to be disrupted in alcohol dependence).
- Not metabolized, cleared as unchanged drug by kidneys; t ½: 20–33 hours.
- No significant drug interactions.

Clinical Pearls:
- Approved by the FDA in 2004, but it has been used in France and other countries since 1989.
- Does not eliminate or treat symptoms of alcohol withdrawal. Usually prescribed for maintenance of abstinence; may continue even if patient relapses with alcohol.
- Clinically, acamprosate has demonstrated efficacy in more than 25 placebo-controlled trials, and has generally been found to be more effective than placebo in reducing risk of returning to any drinking and increasing the cumulative duration of abstinence. However, in reducing heavy drinking, acamprosate appears to be no better than placebo.
- Acamprosate can be used with naltrexone or disulfiram (different mechanism of action), although the combination with naltrexone may not increase efficacy per available studies.
- Taking with food is not necessary, but it may help compliance to do so.
- Compared to naltrexone and disulfiram, acamprosate is unique in that it is not metabolized by the liver and is not impacted by alcohol use, so it can be administered to patients with hepatitis or liver disease and to patients who continue drinking alcohol.

Fun Fact:
Each 333 mg tablet contains 33 mg of elemental calcium (because it is available as acamprosate calcium salt).

Bottom Line:
- Acamprosate and naltrexone show similar reduced rates of relapse, but acamprosate is associated with more diarrhea, while naltrexone is associated with more nausea, fatigue, and somnolence; acamprosate is preferred in patients with hepatic impairment.

BUPRENORPHINE (Buprenex, Probuphine, Sublocade) Fact Sheet [G]

FDA Indications:

Opioid dependence, induction; moderate-severe pain (Belbuca, Buprenex, Butrans). **Opioid dependence, maintenance** (Probuphine).

Dosage Forms:

- **SL tablets (G):** 2 mg, 8 mg (scored).
- **Injection (G):** 0.3 mg/mL (used for pain).
- **Transdermal patch (Butrans):** 5 mcg/h, 7.5 mcg/h, 10 mcg/h, 15 mcg/h, 20 mcg/h (used for pain).
- **Subdermal implant (Probuphine):** Each implant contains equivalent of 80 mg of buprenorphine.
- **Extended release injection (Sublocade):** 100 mg/0.5 mL, 300 mg/1.5 mL prefilled syringes.

Dosage Guidance:

- Start 2 mg–8 mg SL day 1; then 8 mg–16 mg SL QD (usual induction dose range is 12 mg–16 mg/day and accomplished over 3–4 days). Begin at least 4 hours after last use of heroin or other short-acting opioids and when first signs of withdrawal appear. In essence, if an opioid-dependent patient is not in sufficient withdrawal, introduction of buprenorphine may precipitate withdrawal due to its partial agonist effect. Other than implant, not for maintenance treatment; patients should be switched to the buprenorphine/naloxone combination product for maintenance and unsupervised therapy.
- Patients who have been stable on ≤8 mg/day for at least 3 months may convert to implants, available as one-inch-long flexible rods. These rods are surgically implanted on the inside of the upper arm and deliver a low-level dose of buprenorphine for up to 6 months.
- Patients with moderate to severe opioid use disorder and who have been stabilized with SL or buccal buprenorphine for >7 days may convert to monthly injections. Start 300 mg monthly for 2 months, then give 100 mg monthly maintenance doses. Some patients may require higher doses.

Monitoring: No routine monitoring recommended unless clinical picture warrants.

Cost: SL: $$$; implant: $$$$$; monthly injection pricing not yet determined

Side Effects:

- Most common: Headache, pain, insomnia, nausea, anxiety; surgical site pain, itching, redness (Probuphine).
- Serious but rare: Hepatitis reported rarely, ranging from transient, asymptomatic transaminase elevations to hepatic failure; in many cases, patients had preexisting hepatic dysfunction. QT prolongation with higher doses of transdermal patch.

Mechanism, Pharmacokinetics, and Drug Interactions:

- Opioid agonist (delta and mu receptors) and antagonist (kappa receptors).
- Metabolized primarily through CYP3A4; t ½: 24–48 hours.
- Avoid concomitant use with opiate analgesics (diminished pain control). Additive effects with CNS depressants. CYP3A4 inhibitors and inducers may affect levels of buprenorphine.

Clinical Pearls:

- Schedule III controlled substance. Prescribing of SL tablets for opioid dependence is limited to physicians who have met qualification criteria and have received a DEA number specific to buprenorphine (see www.buprenorphine.samhsa.gov).
- Initially, each approved doctor could treat only 10 patients, but the law was modified to alleviate bottlenecks in treatment access; now each physician can treat up to 100 patients and after 1 year can become eligible to treat up to 275.
- Binds to various opioid receptors, producing agonism at delta receptors, partial agonism at mu receptors, and antagonism at kappa receptors (opioid agonist-antagonist).
- Implant and monthly injection offer alternatives that may be convenient for some patients.

Fun Fact:

Other subcutaneous implants currently in development include medications for schizophrenia, breast cancer, photosensitivity, and Parkinson's disease.

Bottom Line:

Buprenorphine alone was previously preferred for the initial (induction) phase of treatment, with buprenorphine/naloxone combination (Suboxone) preferred for maintenance treatment (unsupervised administration). Currently, the combination is favored for both induction and maintenance as this decreases any abuse or diversion potential.

BUPRENORPHINE/NALOXONE (Suboxone) Fact Sheet [G]

FDA Indications:

Opioid dependence (induction and maintenance).

Dosage Forms:

- **SL tablets (G):** 2/0.5 mg, 8/2 mg (scored).
- **SL film strips (Suboxone):** 2/0.5 mg, 4/1 mg, 8/2 mg, 12/3 mg.
- **SL tablets (Zubsolv):** 1.4/0.36 mg, 2.9/0.71 mg, 5.7/1.4 mg, 8.6/2.1 mg, 11.4/2.9 mg.
- **Buccal film (Bunavail):** 2.1/0.3 mg, 4.2/0.7 mg, 6.3/1 mg.

Dosage Guidance:

- For induction, use strategy described in buprenorphine fact sheet. For maintenance, give combination product (Suboxone or [G]) daily in the equivalent buprenorphine dose on last day of induction; adjust dose in increments of 2 mg or 4 mg to a level that maintains treatment and suppresses opioid withdrawal symptoms (usually 4 mg–24 mg/day); max 32 mg/day.
- Zubsolv 5.7/1.4 mg SL tablet provides equivalent buprenorphine to a Suboxone 8/2 mg SL tablet.
- Bunavail 4.2/0.7 mg buccal film provides equivalent buprenorphine to a Suboxone 8/2 mg SL tablet.

Monitoring: No routine monitoring recommended unless clinical picture warrants.

Cost: SL tablet, film: $$$$; Zubsolv, Bunavail: $$$$$

Side Effects:

- Most common: Headache, pain, vomiting, sweating.
- Serious but rare: Hepatitis reported rarely, ranging from transient, asymptomatic transaminase elevations to hepatic failure; in many cases, patients had preexisting hepatic dysfunction.

Mechanism, Pharmacokinetics, and Drug Interactions:

- Buprenorphine: Opioid agonist (delta and mu receptors) and antagonist (kappa receptors); naloxone: Opioid antagonist.
- Metabolized primarily through CYP3A4; t ½: 24–48 hours (naloxone: 2–12 hours).
- Avoid concomitant use with opiate analgesics (diminished pain control). Additive effects with CNS depressants. CYP3A4 inhibitors and inducers may affect levels of buprenorphine.

Clinical Pearls:

- Schedule III controlled substance. Prescribing is limited to physicians who have met qualification criteria and have received a DEA number specific to buprenorphine (see www.buprenorphine.samhsa.gov).
- Naloxone is an opioid antagonist that is active only when injected; it is added to buprenorphine in order to reduce misuse via intravenous injection of a dissolved tablet.
- The SL film formulation's manufacturer claims it dissolves faster and tastes better than SL tablets. Actually, it is more likely a way for the manufacturer to switch users to a "new" product (with patent protection until 2025) rather than lose patients to generics.
- SL film should be placed at base of tongue to the side of midline; this allows patient to use 2 films at the same time if dose dictates.
- Zubsolv and Bunavail formulations have better bioavailability, hence the dose equivalencies noted above.
- Prescribers should be aware of the high risk for diversion and sale of buprenorphine films and tablets. Some regular opioid abusers periodically buy buprenorphine "off the street" and use it to combat cravings and withdrawal symptoms if their drug of choice is not readily available.

Fun Fact:

The manufacturer of Suboxone, Reckitt Benckiser, generates most of its revenue from selling home and personal care products like Lysol cleaners and Durex condoms.

Bottom Line:

The combination product is preferred over buprenorphine alone for maintenance because the addition of naloxone lowers its potential for injection abuse. Although the SL film formulation is currently priced the same as the SL tablets, the SL film strips provide very little (if any) meaningful benefit, and generic SL tablets should be used as a cost-saving measure.

BUPROPION SR (Zyban) Fact Sheet [G]

FDA Indications:
Smoking cessation.

Dosage Forms:
SR tablets (G): 150 mg ER.

Dosage Guidance:
Start 150 mg QAM for 3 days, then 150 mg BID; separate doses by at least 8 hours and administer last dose no later than 6 pm to minimize insomnia. Target smoking quit dates are generally in the second week of treatment.

Monitoring: No routine monitoring recommended unless clinical picture warrants.

Cost: [G]: $; Zyban: $$$$

Side Effects:
- Most common: Agitation, insomnia, headache, nausea, vomiting, tremor, tachycardia, dry mouth, weight loss.
- Serious but rare: Seizures; risk higher with rapid and large dose increases and in patients at risk for seizures. Anaphylactoid reactions (eg, pruritus, urticaria, angioedema, dyspnea) reported rarely; reports include Stevens-Johnson syndrome and anaphylactic shock. Class warning regarding suicide risk (see Antidepressants chapter).

Mechanism, Pharmacokinetics, and Drug Interactions:
- Norepinephrine and dopamine reuptake inhibitor.
- Metabolized primarily through CYP2B6; may inhibit CYP2D6; t ½: 21 hours.
- Avoid use with MAOIs. Levels of drugs metabolized by CYP2D6 (eg, paroxetine, fluoxetine, aripiprazole, iloperidone, atomoxetine, beta blockers) may be increased. Successful cessation of smoking may alter pharmacokinetic properties of other medications (eg, clozapine, olanzapine, theophylline, warfarin, insulin).

Clinical Pearls:
- If patient successfully quits smoking after 7–12 weeks, may consider maintenance therapy based on individual patient risk-benefit. Efficacy of maintenance therapy (150 mg BID) has been shown for up to 6 months. However, if patient has not made significant progress by the seventh week of therapy, success is unlikely and discontinuation should be considered.
- Bupropion slows the weight gain that often occurs in the initial weeks after smoking cessation, but with time, this effect becomes negligible.
- Bupropion and nicotine replacement therapy show similar quit rates: About 25%, or double that seen with placebo, are abstinent at 6 months.
- Equally effective in smokers with or without history of depression.

Fun Fact:
Much of the initial direct-to-consumer advertising that was done for Zyban was via print ads in smoke-free places such as airports.

Bottom Line:
Given the high rate of comorbidity between smoking and depression, this is an attractive intervention for many patients. It is also a particularly good choice for patients who are not able to set a quit date prior to initiating treatment.

DISULFIRAM (Antabuse) Fact Sheet [G]

FDA Indications:
Alcohol dependence.

Dosage Forms:
Tablets (G): 250 mg, 500 mg.

Dosage Guidance:
Start 125 mg QPM (must be abstinent from alcohol >12 hours); increase to 250 mg QPM after several days. Maintenance is usually 250 mg–500 mg QPM, but some patients can drink alcohol without a reaction at the 250 mg/day dose.

Monitoring: Liver function tests if liver disease is suspected.

Cost: $$

Side Effects:
- Most common: Skin eruptions (eg, acne, allergic dermatitis), drowsiness, fatigue, impotence, headache, metallic taste.
- Serious but rare: Severe (very rarely fatal) hepatitis or hepatic failure reported and may occur in patients with or without prior history of abnormal hepatic function. Rare psychotic episodes have been reported. Rarely may cause peripheral neuropathy or optic neuritis.

Mechanism, Pharmacokinetics, and Drug Interactions:
- Aldehyde dehydrogenase inhibitor.
- Metabolized primarily through CYP450; t ½ is not defined, but elimination from body is slow, and effects may persist for 1 or 2 weeks after last dose.
- While taking disulfiram, and for 1–2 weeks after stopping, avoid concomitant use of any medications containing alcohol (including topicals), metronidazole, or "disguised" forms of ethanol (cough syrup, some mouthwashes, oral solutions or liquid concentrates containing alcohol such as sertraline). Avoid vinegars, cider, extracts, and foods containing ethanol.

Clinical Pearls:
- Disulfiram inhibits the enzyme aldehyde dehydrogenase; when taken with alcohol, acetaldehyde levels are increased by 5- to 10-fold, causing unpleasant symptoms that include flushing, nausea, vomiting, palpitations, chest pain, vertigo, hypotension, and (in rare instances) cardiovascular collapse and death. This is the basis for its use as aversion therapy. Common advice to patients: "You'll wish you were dead, but it likely won't kill you."
- Reaction may last from 30–60 minutes to several hours or as long as alcohol remains in the bloodstream.
- Advise patients to carry an identification card or a medical alert bracelet that states they are taking the medication and lists the symptoms of the reaction and clinician contact information.
- Duration of therapy is until the patient is fully recovered and a basis for permanent self-control has been established; maintenance therapy may be required for months or even years.

Fun Fact:
Disulfiram's anti-protozoal activity may be effective in *Giardia* and *Trichomonas* infections.

Bottom Line:
Since craving is not reduced by disulfiram and any alcohol ingestion could result in a reaction, noncompliance can be common. Its use should be reserved for selective, highly motivated patients in conjunction with supportive and psychotherapeutic treatment.

METHADONE (Methadose) Fact Sheet [G]

FDA Indications:

Opioid dependence; severe pain.

Dosage Forms:

- **Tablets (G):** 5 mg, 10 mg, 40 mg (scored),
- **Oral solution (G):** 10 mg/5 mL, 5 mg/5 mL.
- **Oral concentrate (G):** 10 mg/mL.

Dosage Guidance:

Start 15 mg–30 mg single dose; then 5 mg–10 mg every 2–4 hours. Adjust dose to prevent withdrawal symptoms; max 40 mg on day 1. 80 mg–120 mg per day is a common maintenance dose for opioid dependence.

Monitoring: ECG if cardiac disease.

Cost: $

Side Effects:

- Most common: Constipation, dizziness, sedation, nausea, sweating.
- Serious but rare: May prolong the QTc interval and increase risk for torsades de pointes; caution in patients at risk for QTc prolongation; usually with doses >100 mg/day. Severe respiratory depression may occur; use extreme caution during initiation, titration, and conversion from other opiates to methadone. Respiratory depressant effects occur later and persist longer than analgesic effects, possibly contributing to cases of overdose.

Mechanism, Pharmacokinetics, and Drug Interactions:

- Opioid agonist.
- Metabolized primarily through CYP2B6, 2C19, and 3A4 (major); inhibits CYP2D6; t ½: 8–59 hours.
- High potential for interactions. Avoid concomitant use with other potent sedatives or respiratory depressants. Use with caution in patients on medications that are metabolized by CYP2D6, inhibit CYP3A4, prolong the QTc interval, or promote electrolyte depletion.

Clinical Pearls:

- Schedule II controlled substance; distribution of 40 mg tablets restricted to authorized opioid addiction treatment facilities.
- May only be dispensed according to the Substance Abuse and Mental Health Services Administration's (SAMHSA) Center for Substance Abuse Treatment (CSAT) guidelines. Regulations vary by area; consult regulatory agencies and/or methadone treatment facilities.
- Methadone accumulates with repeated doses; dose may need reduction after 3–5 days to prevent CNS depressant effects.

Fun Fact:

A persistent but untrue urban legend claims the name "Dolophine" was coined in tribute to Adolf Hitler by its German creators. The name was in fact created after the war by the American branch of Eli Lilly, and the pejorative term "adolphine" (never an actual name of the drug) didn't appear in the US until the early 1970s.

Bottom Line:

Opiate replacement therapy via methadone reduces or eliminates illicit use of opiates and criminality associated with opiate use, allowing patients to improve health and social functioning. It is a successful harm reduction model because it reduces the transmission of infectious diseases associated with opiate injection, such as hepatitis and HIV. Disadvantages include potential for accumulation with repeated doses (which may result in toxicity), interindividual variability in pharmacokinetic parameters, potential for drug interactions, challenges associated with dose titration, stigma associated with opiate replacement therapy, and limited availability of treatment programs (eg, nonexistent in some geographic areas, long wait lists in other areas).

NALOXONE (Evzio, Narcan Nasal Spray) Fact Sheet [G]

FDA Indications:

Emergency treatment of known or suspected opioid overdose.

Dosage Forms:

- **Pre-filled auto-injector (Evzio):** 2 mg/0.4 mL.
- **Intranasal (Narcan Nasal Spray):** 4 mg/0.1 mL.
- Generic intranasal kit may be assembled using 2 mg/2 mL prefilled needleless syringe and a mucosal atomization device nasal adapter (requires assembly at time of administration).

Dosage Guidance:

- Auto-injector: Bystander to administer 2 mg IM into thigh, through clothing if necessary as directed by voice prompt; may repeat with additional doses every 2–3 minutes if no or minimal response and until emergency response arrives.
- Intranasal: Bystander to spray in one nostril; may repeat into other nostril with additional doses every 2–3 minutes if no or minimal response and until emergency response arrives.

Monitoring: No routine monitoring recommended unless clinical picture warrants.

Cost: Auto-injector: $$$$$; intranasal: $$$; generic kit: $

Side Effects:

- Most common: Symptoms of opioid withdrawal, including body aches, fever, sweating, runny nose, sneezing, piloerection, yawning, weakness, shivering or trembling, nervousness, restlessness or irritability, diarrhea, nausea or vomiting, abdominal cramps, increased blood pressure, and tachycardia.

Mechanism, Pharmacokinetics, and Drug Interactions:

- Opioid antagonist.
- Metabolized primarily by conjugation (non-P450) in the liver; t ½: 1.36 hours.

Clinical Pearls:

- Because treatment of overdose with this opioid antagonist must be performed by someone other than the patient, instruct prescription recipients to inform those around them that they have naloxone rescue and ensure that those people have been instructed in recognizing overdose symptoms and how to administer the medication.
- Evzio comes with printed instructions on the device label as well as electronic voice instructions (there is a speaker that provides instructions to guide the user through each step of the injection).
- Most opioids have a longer duration of action than naloxone, so it's likely that overdose symptoms (CNS depression and respiratory depression) will return after initial improvement. Therefore, patients should continue to be monitored and should receive medical attention after emergency dose(s) provided.
- Intranasal forms of naloxone rescue administration, if broadly distributed to those at risk, could make overdose rescue a more acceptable and widespread practice.
- Check out the Prescribe to Prevent website (prescribetoprevent.org) for prescriber resources such as webinars, toolkits, patient education materials, and medical-legal resources. This website also provides guidance to physicians on writing a prescription for naloxone.

Fun Fact:

Naloxone was first approved for opioid overdose treatment in 1971 and is available as a very inexpensive injectable generic. These newer formulations will come at a much higher price because of the way they are formulated, making them easier to use by non-emergency provider bystanders.

Bottom Line:

Naloxone rescue saves lives. Prescribe it.

NALTREXONE (ReVia, Vivitrol) Fact Sheet [G]

FDA Indications:
Alcohol dependence; opioid addiction (relapse prevention following detox).

Off-Label Uses:
Self-injurious behavior.

Dosage Forms:
- **Tablets (ReVia, G):** 50 mg (scored).
- **Long-acting injection (Vivitrol):** 380 mg.

Dosage Guidance:
- Opioid dependence: Start 25 mg for 1 day; if no withdrawal signs, increase to and maintain 50 mg/day (with food); doses >50 mg may increase risk of hepatotoxicity.
- Alcohol dependence: Start and maintain 50 mg QD.
- Injection: 380 mg IM (gluteal) Q4 weeks (for opioid or alcohol dependence). Do not initiate therapy until patient is opioid-free for at least 7–10 days (by urinalysis).

Monitoring: Liver function tests if liver disease is suspected.

Cost: Tablet: $; injection: $$$$$

Side Effects:
- Most common: Headache, nausea, somnolence, vomiting.
- Serious but rare: Black box warning regarding dose-related hepatocellular injury; the difference between apparent safe and hepatotoxic doses appears to be ≤5-fold (narrow therapeutic window). Discontinue if signs/symptoms of acute hepatitis develop.

Mechanism, Pharmacokinetics, and Drug Interactions:
- Opioid antagonist.
- Metabolized primarily through non-CYP450 pathway; t ½: 4 hours (5–10 days for IM).
- No significant interactions other than avoiding use with opiates (see below).

Clinical Pearls:
- May precipitate acute withdrawal (pain, hypertension, sweating, agitation, and irritability) in opiate-using patients; ensure patient is opioid-free for at least 7–10 days prior to initiating.
- In naltrexone-treated patients requiring emergency pain management, consider alternatives to opiates (eg, regional analgesia, non-opioid analgesics, general anesthesia). If opioid therapy is required, patients should be under the direct care of a trained anesthesia provider.
- Efficacy of oral naltrexone in alcohol dependence (craving and relapse) is more convincing than in opiate dependence. In opiate dependence, craving is not decreased but euphoric effects are blocked. Monthly IM naltrexone may be more effective than oral at maintaining abstinence in opiate dependence, without concern for daily medication adherence.

Fun Fact:
Methylnaltrexone, a closely related drug, is marketed as Relistor for the treatment of opioid-induced constipation.

Bottom Line:
Naltrexone is more frequently used for alcohol dependence than for opiate dependence. It is often used to minimize severity of drinking, while acamprosate is used to prevent relapse. Avoid naltrexone in patients with hepatic impairment or those taking opiate-based pain medications. For opioid dependence, methadone and buprenorphine are more effective for most, although naltrexone may be appropriate for highly motivated opiate-dependent patients, with injectable preferred over oral.

NICOTINE GUM/LOZENGE (Nicorette) Fact Sheet [G]

FDA Indications:
Smoking cessation.

Dosage Forms:
- **Gum (G):** 2 mg, 4 mg (over the counter).
- **Lozenge (G):** 2 mg, 4 mg (over the counter).

Dosage Guidance:
- For gum: Chew 1 piece of gum PRN urge to smoke, up to 24 pieces/day. Patients who smoke <25 cigarettes/day should start with the 2 mg strength; patients smoking ≥25 cigarettes/day should start with the 4 mg strength. Use the following 12-week dosing schedule: For weeks 1–6, chew 1 piece of gum every 1–2 hours; to increase chances of quitting, chew at least 9 pieces/day. For weeks 7–9, chew 1 piece of gum every 2–4 hours. For weeks 10–12, chew 1 piece of gum every 4–8 hours. Patients should not chew more than 1 piece of gum at a time.
- For lozenges: Patients who smoke their first cigarette within 30 minutes of waking should use the 4 mg strength; otherwise the 2 mg strength is recommended. Use the following 12-week dosing schedule: For weeks 1–6, use 1 lozenge every 1–2 hours; to increase chances of quitting, use at least 9 lozenges/day. For weeks 7–9, use 1 lozenge every 2–4 hours. For weeks 10–12, use 1 lozenge every 4–8 hours. Maximum dose is 5 lozenges every 6 hours or 20 lozenges/day. Patients should not use more than 1 lozenge at a time.
- Patients should be advised to completely stop smoking upon initiation of therapy.

Monitoring: No routine monitoring recommended unless clinical picture warrants.

Cost: $

Side Effects:
Most common: Headache; indigestion; nausea; hiccups; tongue, mouth, and throat irritation or tingling; jaw ache (gum).

Mechanism, Pharmacokinetics, and Drug Interactions:
- Nicotinic-cholinergic receptor agonist.
- Metabolized primarily through liver as well as kidneys and lungs; t ½: 1–2 hours.
- Minimal risk for drug interactions. Successful cessation of smoking may increase serum levels of medications metabolized by CYP1A2 (eg, clozapine, olanzapine, theophylline), which is induced by hydrocarbons in smoke; nicotine itself has no effect.

Clinical Pearls:
- Chew gum slowly until it tingles (about 15 chews), then park gum between cheek and gum until tingle is gone (about 1 minute); repeat until most of tingle is gone (~30 minutes).
- Lozenges should not be chewed or swallowed; allow them to dissolve slowly (~20–30 minutes).
- Heavy smokers should use higher-dose gum or lozenge and at least 9 pieces/day to maximize chances of success. Do not use more than 1 piece at a time.
- Each 4 mg lozenge or gum results in 2 mg of absorbed nicotine, equivalent to 2 cigarettes.

Fun Fact:
Nicotine gum is available in a variety of flavors (fruit, mint, cinnamon, orange, cherry, and "original").

Bottom Line:
First-line intervention for those patients who can stop smoking at initiation of therapy; nicotine in the form of gum or lozenge may act as a substitute oral activity, which may aid in behavior modification.

NICOTINE INHALED (Nicotrol Inhaler) Fact Sheet

FDA Indications:
Smoking cessation.

Dosage Forms:
Cartridge: 4 mg delivered per 10 mg cartridge (prescription required).

Dosage Guidance:

- Use frequent continuous puffing for 20 minutes with each cartridge; 80 deep inhalations over 20 minutes releases 4 mg nicotine, of which 2 mg is absorbed. Use 6–16 cartridges per day. Taper after 6–12 weeks of use by gradual dose reduction over 6–12 additional weeks.
- Patients should be advised to completely stop smoking upon initiation of therapy.

Monitoring: No routine monitoring recommended unless clinical picture warrants.

Cost: $$$$

Side Effects:
Most common: Headache, mouth/throat irritation, dyspepsia, cough, unpleasant taste, rhinitis, tearing, sneezing.

Mechanism, Pharmacokinetics, and Drug Interactions:

- Nicotinic-cholinergic receptor agonist.
- Metabolized primarily through liver as well as kidneys and lungs; t ½: 1–2 hours.
- Minimal risk for drug interactions. Successful cessation of smoking may increase serum levels of medications metabolized by CYP1A2 (eg, clozapine, olanzapine, theophylline), which is induced by hydrocarbons in smoke; nicotine itself has no effect.

Clinical Pearls:

- Insert cartridge into inhaler and push hard until it pops into place. Replace mouthpiece and twist the top and bottom so that markings do not line up. Inhale deeply into the back of the throat or puff in short breaths. Nicotine in cartridge is used up after about 20 minutes of active puffing.
- Do not eat or drink 15 minutes before or during use. Puff lightly rather than inhale into lungs to minimize coughing.
- Local irritation in the mouth and throat may occur in as many as 40% of patients; coughing (32%) and rhinitis (23%) are also common. These effects are generally mild and occur less frequently with continued use. Use with caution in patients with bronchospastic disease due to potential airway irritation (other forms of nicotine replacement may be preferred).
- Higher ambient temperatures deliver more nicotine; lower temperatures deliver less.
- 1 cartridge delivers 80 puffs or about 2 mg of absorbed nicotine. Roughly 10 cartridges per day is equivalent to the nicotine of smoking 1 pack per day.

Fun Fact:
A nicotine inhaler is not really a true inhaler; puffing deposits the nicotine into the mouth, and it is then absorbed in the same manner as the nicotine gum or lozenge preparations.

Bottom Line:
Very high expense and unpleasant side effects make this form of nicotine replacement therapy difficult to recommend as a first-line option since no single therapy has been shown to be more effective than another.

NICOTINE NASAL SPRAY (Nicotrol NS) Fact Sheet

FDA Indications:
Smoking cessation.

Dosage Forms:
10 mL bottle: 10 mg/mL delivering 0.5 mg/spray in 200 sprays (prescription required).

Dosage Guidance:
- Use 1–2 sprays/hour as needed; do not exceed more than 5 doses (10 sprays) per hour. Max dose is 40 doses/day (80 sprays). Each dose (2 sprays) contains 1 mg of nicotine.
- After initial 8 weeks of treatment, taper dose gradually over 4–6 weeks.
- Patients should be advised to completely stop smoking upon initiation of therapy.

Monitoring: No routine monitoring recommended unless clinical picture warrants.

Cost: $$$$

Side Effects:
Most common: Headache, dyspepsia, rhinitis, nasal irritation, sneezing, coughing.

Mechanism, Pharmacokinetics, and Drug Interactions:
- Nicotinic-cholinergic receptor agonist.
- Metabolized primarily through liver as well as kidneys and lungs; t ½: 1–2 hours.
- Minimal risk for drug interactions. Successful cessation of smoking may increase serum levels of medications metabolized by CYP1A2 (eg, clozapine, olanzapine, theophylline), which is induced by hydrocarbons in smoke; nicotine itself has no effect.

Clinical Pearls:
- Prime pump prior to first use. Blow nose gently prior to use. Tilt head back slightly, breathe through mouth, and spray once in each nostril. Do not sniff, swallow, or inhale through nose.
- Moderate to severe nasal irritation in 94% of patients in the first 2 days of use; severity decreases over time. Nasal congestion and transient changes in sense of smell and taste also reported. Avoid in patients with chronic nasal disorders (eg, allergy, rhinitis, nasal polyps, and sinusitis). Exacerbations of bronchospasm reported in patients with asthma.
- Heavy smokers may well use the maximum amount of 80 sprays/day, meaning they would need a new bottle every 2–3 days. This can be tremendously and prohibitively expensive.
- Potential for abuse and dependence appears to be greater than with other NRT.

Fun Fact:
In a published case report (*Am J Psychiatry* 2001), a 54-year-old man who could no longer afford his Nicotrol NS prescription found a commercial source for nicotine on the internet (sold as an insecticide). He purchased 25 g in a 1 g/mL solution for $30, diluted the nicotine solution with distilled water to 10 mg/mL, and then placed the solution into empty spray bottles.

Bottom Line:
The idea of nasal administration of nicotine is appealing in that it more closely approximates the time course of plasma nicotine levels observed after cigarette smoking than other dosage forms; however, the high cost coupled with unpleasant side effects make this difficult to recommend as a first-line treatment, especially since no one form of nicotine replacement therapy has been shown to be more effective than another.

NICOTINE PATCH (Nicoderm CQ) Fact Sheet [G]

FDA Indications:
Smoking cessation.

Dosage Forms:
Transdermal patch (G): 7 mg, 14 mg, 21 mg/24 hour (over the counter).

Dosage Guidance:
- Apply new patch every 24 hours (same time each day, usually after awakening) to non-hairy, clean, dry skin on the upper body or upper outer arm; each patch should be applied to a different site. Adjustment may be required during initial treatment (move to higher dose if experiencing withdrawal symptoms, or lower dose if side effects are experienced). Patients smoking >10 cigarettes/day: Start with 21 mg/day for 6 weeks, then 14 mg/day for 2 weeks, then 7 mg/day for 2 weeks. Patients smoking ≤10 cigarettes/day: Start with 14 mg/day for 6 weeks, then 7 mg/day for 2 weeks.
- Patients should be advised to completely stop smoking upon initiation of therapy.

Monitoring: No routine monitoring recommended unless clinical picture warrants.

Cost: $

Side Effects:
- Most common: Application site reactions (itching, burning, or redness), diarrhea, dyspepsia, abdominal pain.

Mechanism, Pharmacokinetics, and Drug Interactions:
- Nicotinic-cholinergic receptor agonist.
- Metabolized primarily through liver as well as kidneys and lungs; t ½: 3–6 hours.
- Minimal risk for drug interactions. Successful cessation of smoking may increase serum levels of medications metabolized by CYP1A2 (eg, clozapine, olanzapine, theophylline), which is induced by hydrocarbons in smoke; nicotine itself has no effect.

Clinical Pearls:
- Patch may be worn for 16 or 24 hours. If craving upon awakening, wear patch for 24 hours; if vivid dreams or sleep disruptions occur, wear patch for 16 hours, removing at bedtime.
- Do not cut patch; this causes rapid evaporation, making the patch useless.
- Up to 50% of patients will experience a local skin reaction, which is usually mild and self-limiting but may worsen with continued treatment. Local treatment with hydrocortisone cream 1% or triamcinolone cream 0.5% and rotating patch sites may help. In fewer than 5% of patients, such reactions require discontinuation.

Fun Facts:
Studies have found that smoking seems to provide short-term relief from symptoms of ulcerative colitis; recent data have suggested the use of nicotine patches in some patients with flare-ups of ulcerative colitis (not maintenance treatment).

Bottom Line:
Nicotine patches are a first-line intervention in patients who are able to quit smoking at initiation of treatment and who are regular and constant smokers.

VARENICLINE (Chantix) Fact Sheet

FDA Indications:
Smoking cessation.

Dosage Forms:
Tablets: 0.5 mg, 1 mg.

Dosage Guidance:
Start 0.5 mg QD for 3 days; ↑ to 0.5 mg BID for 4 days then ↑ to 1 mg BID for 11 weeks. Titrate slowly and take with food and a full glass of water to decrease GI upset. Start 1 week before target quit date; consider setting a quit date up to 35 days after starting varenicline (may improve likelihood of abstinence).

Monitoring: No routine monitoring recommended unless clinical picture warrants.

Cost: $$$$

Side Effects:
- Most common: Nausea, insomnia, headache, abnormal dreams, constipation, flatulence.
- Serious but rare: Warning for serious neuropsychiatric events (including depression, suicidal thoughts, suicide, psychosis, hostility), even in those without preexisting psychiatric disease, was recently revised to indicate that risk is lower than previously suspected.

Mechanism, Pharmacokinetics, and Drug Interactions:
- Nicotine receptor partial agonist.
- Excreted mostly unchanged with minimal hepatic (non-CYP450) metabolism; t ½: 24 hours.
- Potential lowered tolerance to alcohol, with psychiatric reactions. H2 blockers, quinolones, and trimethoprim may increase varenicline levels. Successful cessation of smoking may alter pharmacokinetic properties of other medications (eg, clozapine, olanzapine, theophylline, warfarin, insulin).

Clinical Pearls:
- Dual mechanism of action: Partial agonist at nicotinic receptors, mimicking nicotine effects on the brain and reducing withdrawal symptoms; blocks nicotine from binding to these receptors, thereby decreasing the reinforcing effect of smoking.
- If patient successfully quits smoking after 12 weeks, may continue for another 12 weeks. If not successful in first 12 weeks, then discontinue and reassess factors contributing to failure.
- Similar quit rates as bupropion at 6 months (25%), but higher quit rates compared to bupropion at 1 year if a second 12-week course of varenicline is used.
- Can be combined with bupropion; use with nicotine replacement therapies likely to lead to increased side effects, particularly nausea, headache, vomiting, and dizziness.

Fun Fact:
The show *Saturday Night Live* aired a parody of a Chantix commercial suggesting that side effects of *quitting* smoking could be dangerous (it's on YouTube).

Bottom Line:
Varenicline is the most effective tobacco cessation medication. Psychiatric side effects are usually limited to insomnia or abnormal dreams, but more dramatic reactions are possible, though rare.

Appendices

APPENDIX A: DRUG INTERACTIONS IN PSYCHIATRY

Drug interactions can be one of the most challenging aspects of psychopharmacology. Today's psychiatrists often use complex medication regimens, while patients frequently take drugs for multiple medical comorbidities. It's impossible to keep track of all of these, but it is important (1) to understand basic concepts of drug-drug interactions, (2) to know where to find information regarding such interactions, and (3) to know which interactions may be clinically relevant.

The majority of interactions in psychiatry will not result in a serious outcome. Many interactions, however, may result in decreased efficacy or increased adverse effects, and these can be easily avoided.

First, let's review some basic concepts. A drug interaction occurs when the pharmacologic action of one drug is altered by the coadministration of another drug. The two major types of drug interactions are **pharmacodynamic** (what the drug does to the body) and **pharmacokinetic** (what the body does to the drug). Pharmacodynamic interactions impact the effects of the drug at the target site. Pharmacokinetic interactions, on the other hand, impact the amount of time the drug stays in the body and its distribution to active sites.

Pharmacodynamic interactions take place at the level of neurotransmitters and receptors. For example, clonazepam (Klonopin) makes people sleepy by stimulating GABA receptors. Quetiapine (Seroquel) also makes people sleepy, probably by blocking histamine receptors. Combine the two, and patients become *really* sleepy. Pharmacodynamic interactions may also cause two drugs to *oppose* one another. Many of the dementia medications, for example, increase acetylcholine levels, while many psychiatric medications have primary (eg, benztropine) or secondary (eg, clozapine) anticholinergic effects. Giving both together may negate the beneficial effects of the dementia medication.

Some notable—and potentially dangerous—pharmacodynamic interactions in psychiatry include serotonin syndrome (too many serotonergic agents used together); the MAOI-type hypertensive crisis (MAOIs taken with foods high in tyramine); and arrhythmia-causing combinations (medications that increase QT interval, when taken together, may cause life-threatening arrhythmias, such as torsades de pointes). We often try to avoid these problems by doing things like lowering doses or choosing alternative medications. In such cases, we're trying to avoid pharmacodynamic interactions.

Pharmacokinetic interactions are harder to predict, since they are non-intuitive and are unrelated to the pharmacologic action of drugs. Pharmacokinetic interactions depend on where and when two or more drugs come in contact during drug processing. Drugs can interact with one another at four different junctures:

- Absorption (getting the drug into the bloodstream)
- Distribution (ferrying drugs to different tissues once they've been absorbed)
- Excretion (sending drugs into the sewage system)
- Metabolism (dismantling drugs into simpler components)

We'll discuss each one in turn, focusing on some common examples in psychopharmacology.

Absorption. Drug-food, rather than drug-drug, interactions are most relevant during absorption. For example, ziprasidone (Geodon) and lurasidone (Latuda) absorption is decreased by 50%–60% when taken without food, which is why we instruct our patients to take these drugs after a full meal (at least, we *should* be doing this!). Food also speeds absorption of both sertraline (Zoloft) and quetiapine, but only by 25% or so, usually not enough to be clinically relevant. Meanwhile, food famously *slows* absorption of erectile dysfunction drugs such as sildenafil (Viagra) and vardenafil (Levitra)—but not tadalafil (Cialis).

Distribution. Valproic acid (Depakote) is highly protein bound, and only the unbound portion (the "free fraction") of the drug has a therapeutic effect. Aspirin is also highly protein bound, so if your patient combines the two drugs, the aspirin will kick some of the valproic acid off its protein—mainly albumin—which would cause the free fraction of the drug to increase. Standard valproic acid levels in the lab usually do not distinguish between free and bound fractions, so a serum level might be normal, even though the actual functioning valproic acid can be very high—and this could potentially cause side effects. One way to check for this interaction is to order a free valproate level; the normal therapeutic range is about 5 mcg/mL–10 mcg/mL, much less than the total valproic acid therapeutic range of about 40 mcg/mL–100 mcg/mL.

Excretion. Lithium, unlike almost all other drugs in psychiatry, is not metabolized. Instead, it is excreted unchanged in the urine. Because of this, liver disease does not affect lithium levels, but changes in kidney function will affect such levels. Caffeine, for example, speeds up kidney function and can reduce lithium levels. On the other hand, ibuprofen (along with other NSAIDs) and ACE inhibitors decrease lithium excretion, increase lithium levels, and could potentially cause toxic effects. Other psychiatric medications that are not metabolized by the liver and rather excreted by the kidneys are gabapentin (Neurontin), pregabalin (Lyrica), and paliperidone (Invega).

Liver metabolism. Most drug-drug interactions take place in the liver, where drugs are processed in order to render them water soluble so that the body can excrete them via the urine or feces. There are two phases of liver metabolism. Phase I involves the famous cytochrome P-450 enzymes, or CYP450. These enzymes attack drugs in a variety of ways, such as hydroxylation (adding a hydroxyl group), dealkylation (taking away an alkyl group), and several others. Unfortunately for those of us trying to remember drug interactions, there are many subfamilies of CYP450 enzymes: CYP1A2, 2B6, 2C9, 2C19, 2D6, 3A4, and several others. Phase II metabolism continues the process of biotransformation, relying mainly on glucuronidation—which is rarely a factor in drug interactions in psychiatric practice.

Practical Implications of Drug-Drug Interactions

To understand drug-drug interactions, you'll need to refamiliarize yourself with some basic terms. Drugs are **substrates** of specific enzymes (the medication relies on that/those enzymatic pathway(s) for metabolism). An **inhibitor** is a drug that binds more tightly to an enzyme than the usual substrate and prevents the enzyme from doing its job; as a result, the substrate for that enzyme gets stuck in a game of musical chairs as it scurries around looking for a free enzyme system to break it down. Since this drug is not getting metabolized as quickly as it otherwise would (the inhibitor is preventing it from doing so), its serum levels become higher than expected. On the other hand, **inducers** stimulate the production of extra enzymes. With more enzymes around, the substrate for that enzyme is broken down more rapidly, leading to lower serum drug levels.

Now that you know the basics, how can you most efficiently apply them to your practice? Here are some suggestions.

- Identify the 10 drugs that you most commonly prescribe, and memorize the major drug interactions for each one.
- Antidepressants, antipsychotics, antibiotics, antiretrovirals, and older anticonvulsants have a high likelihood of significant drug interactions—so be particularly vigilant if your patient is taking any of these.
- Recognize the drugs with a narrow therapeutic window, ie, when the toxic dose is not much higher than the therapeutic dose. Commonly used drugs with narrow therapeutic windows include lithium, carbamazepine (Tegretol), warfarin (Coumadin), digoxin (Lanoxin), phenytoin (Dilantin), and phenobarbital.
- Recognize drugs that cause serious side effects and outcomes if blood levels are significantly increased or decreased (eg, oral contraceptives, lamotrigine, clozapine, TCAs, warfarin).
- Drugs with long half-lives, such as diazepam (Valium) or aripiprazole (Abilify), can be particularly troublesome when involved in drug interactions, because metabolic inhibitors—or hepatic dysfunction—can make them ultra long lasting. Be cautious with any new or rarely prescribed drugs: Neither you nor anybody else has had much experience with them, and unreported drug interactions can appear.
- The risk of drug interactions can increase exponentially as the number of drugs increases. Setting a threshold to check for interactions is helpful (eg, any patient on 3 or more drugs).

Another important concern with drug interactions is timing. *Inhibition* happens quickly. It can occur with the first dose of a medication and can subside quickly. How long it takes to subside depends on the inhibitor's half-life. Generally, the inhibition will stop after 5 half-lives of the inhibitor drug. On the other hand, for *induction* to occur, the body has to synthesize more CYP450 enzymes, and this can take up to 4 weeks. This accounts for the delayed "auto-induction" of carbamazepine. Likewise, for induction to subside, these extra enzymes need to be broken down, a process that could also take several weeks. As a general rule of thumb, any drug prescribed with its inhibitor should be started at half the usual dose and titrated more slowly. Conversely, a drug prescribed with its inducer may need to be dosed higher after the few weeks it takes for induction to occur.

Useful References for Drug Interactions

It's ideal to have a useful resource to look up interaction information. Keeping track of interactions has become less daunting with the advent of free software from companies like Epocrates (www.epocrates.com) and Medscape (www.medscape.com), which allow you to check for potential interactions among all possible combinations of drugs.

But there are various problems with the computerized databases you'll find at these sites or in your electronic prescribing system (if you have one). For one, the databases tend to be overly inclusive, often listing every conceivable interaction, no matter how unlikely. As an example, citalopram (Celexa), an SSRI considered by most of us to be a pretty safe choice in combination with just about any drug, looks pretty dangerous in the Epocrates database. Moreover, these databases are often populated with drug-class information rather than medication-specific information, making important nuances unavailable to the user. That's where your clinical judgment and experience come in!

Free

- Medscape (www.medscape.com/druginfo/druginterchecker)
- http://www.epocrates.com/(you'll need to register first)
- https://www.drugs.com/drug_interactions.html
- http://medicine.iupui.edu/clinpharm/ddis

Not free

- Lexi-Interact (http://bit.ly/fugKmk), $75 1-year subscription

We also provide a table, CYP450 Drug Interactions for Some Commonly Prescribed Medications, on the following pages for your reference (adapted from Goren J & Carlat D, *The Carlat Psychiatry Report* 2011;9(2):1–5).

APPENDIX A TABLE: CYP450 Drug Interactions for Some Commonly Prescribed Medications

CYP450 Family	Inducers	Inhibitors	Substrates ("Victim" Drugs)	Symptoms When Induced	Symptoms When Inhibited
1A2	Armodafinil Carbamazepine Cigarette smoke Modafinil Omeprazole Rifampin Ritonavir St. John's wort	Ciprofloxacin Fluvoxamine Melatonin Norfloxacin	Asenapine	Loss of efficacy (psychosis)	Insomnia/EPS
			Caffeine	Withdrawal headaches	Jitteriness
			Clozapine	Loss of efficacy (psychosis)	Seizures/sedation/anticholinergic effects
			Duloxetine	Loss of efficacy (depression)	Increased blood pressure
			Fluvoxamine	Loss of efficacy (depression/OCD)	GI/sedation
			Melatonin	Loss of efficacy (insomnia)	Sedation
			Mirtazapine	Loss of efficacy (depression)	Sedation
			Olanzapine	Loss of efficacy (psychosis)	Sedation
			Ramelteon	Loss of efficacy (insomnia)	Sedation
			Tasimelteon	Loss of efficacy (insomnia)	Sedation
			Thiothixene	Loss of efficacy (psychosis)	EPS
			Trifluoperazine	Loss of efficacy (psychosis)	EPS
2B6	Carbamazepine Phenobarbital Phenytoin Rifampin	Clopidogrel Ketoconazole Ticlopidine	Bupropion	Loss of efficacy (depression)	Seizures/jitteriness/insomnia
			Methadone	Opiate withdrawal	CNS and respiratory depression
			Selegiline	Loss of efficacy (depression)	Insomnia/diarrhea
2C9	Barbiturates Carbamazepine Rifampin St. John's wort	Fluconazole Fluoxetine Fluvoxamine Isoniazid Metronidazole	Methadone	Opiate withdrawal	CNS and respiratory depression
			NSAIDs	Loss of pain control	GI effects
			Oral hypoglycemics	Loss of glycemic control	Hypoglycemia
			Warfarin	Loss of anticoagulant efficacy	Increased bleeding
2C19	Barbiturates Carbamazepine Rifampin	Fluconazole Fluoxetine Fluvoxamine Modafinil Oxcarbazepine	Barbiturates	Loss of efficacy (insomnia/anxiety/seizures)	Sedation/barb intoxication
			Citalopram	Loss of efficacy (depression/anxiety)	GI effects
			Diazepam	Loss of efficacy (insomnia/anxiety/seizures)	Sedation/BZD intoxication
			Doxepin	Loss of efficacy (depression/anxiety/ insomnia)	Seizures/arrhythmia/anticholinergic effects
			Escitalopram	Loss of efficacy (depression/anxiety)	GI effects
			Methadone	Opiate withdrawal	CNS and respiratory depression
			Sertraline	Loss of efficacy (depression/anxiety)	GI effects

CYP450 Family	Inducers	Inhibitors	Substrates ("Victim" Drugs)	Symptoms When Induced	Symptoms When Inhibited
2D6	Not inducible	Asenapine Bupropion Duloxetine Fluoxetine Haloperidol Methadone Paroxetine (Perphenazine) Thioridazine Venlafaxine	Amphetamine	N/A	Insomnia/decreased appetite
			Aripiprazole	N/A	Akathisia/sedation
			Atomoxetine	N/A	GI/constipation
			Brexpiprazole	N/A	Akathisia/sedation
			Chlorpromazine	N/A	Seizures/sedation/anticholinergic effects
			Clozapine	N/A	Seizures/sedation/anticholinergic effects
			Codeine/hydrocodone	N/A	Less/no analgesia (not converted to morphine)
			Dextroamphetamine	N/A	Insomnia/decreased appetite
			Diphenhydramine	N/A	Sedation/anticholinergic
			Donepezil	N/A	GI effects
			Doxepin	N/A	Sedation/anticholinergic
			Doxylamine	N/A	Sedation/anticholinergic
			Duloxetine	N/A	Increased BP
			Fluoxetine	N/A	GI effects
			Fluphenazine	N/A	EPS
			Fluvoxamine	N/A	GI effects/sedation
			Galantamine	N/A	GI effects
			Haloperidol	N/A	EPS
			Iloperidone	N/A	Tachycardia/hypotension/stiffness
			Loxapine	N/A	EPS/sedation
			Methamphetamine	N/A	Insomnia/decreased appetite
			Mirtazapine	N/A	Somnolence
			Mixed amphetamine salts	N/A	Insomnia/decreased appetite
			Paroxetine	N/A	GI effects/anticholinergic/sedation
			Perphenazine	N/A	EPS/sedation
			Propranolol	N/A	Decreased BP/pulse
			Risperidone	N/A	EPS/orthostasis
			Thioridazine	N/A	Seizures/sedation/anticholinergic effects/ QT prolongation
			Trazodone	N/A	Sedation
			Tricyclics	N/A	Seizures/arrhythmia/anticholinergic
			Venlafaxine	N/A	GIeffects
			Vortioxetine	N/A	GI effects

CYP450 Family	Inducers	Inhibitors	Substrates ("Victim" Drugs)	Symptoms When Induced	Symptoms When Inhibited
3A4	Armodafinil Barbiturates Carbamazepine Modafinil Oxcarbazepine Phenytoin Rifampin St. John's wort (Topiramate)	Clarithromycin Fluconazole Fluvoxamine Grapefruit juice Ketoconazole Protease inhibitors	Alprazolam	Loss of efficacy (insomnia/anxiety/seizures)	Sedation/BZD intoxication
			Aripiprazole	Loss of efficacy (psychosis)	Akathisia/sedation
			Armodafinil	Loss of efficacy (narcolepsy)	Insomnia/increased pulse
			Avanafil	Loss of efficacy (sexual dysfunction)	Headache/flushing/prolonged erection
			Brexpiprazole	Loss of efficacy (psychosis)	Akathisia/sedation
			Buprenorphine	Opiate withdrawal	CNS and respiratory depression
			Buspirone	Loss of efficacy (anxiety)	GI effects/jitteriness
			Calcium channel blockers	Loss of efficacy (hypertension)	Hypotension
			Carbamazepine	Loss of efficacy/seizures	Sedation/arrhythmia
			Cariprazine	Loss of efficacy (psychosis)	Akathisia/sedation
			Citalopram	Loss of efficacy (depression/anxiety)	GI effects
			Clonazepam	Loss of efficacy (insomnia/anxiety/seizures)	Sedation/BZD intoxication
			Clozapine	Loss of efficacy (psychosis)	Seizures/sedation/anticholinergic effects
			Diazepam	Loss of efficacy (insomnia/anxiety/seizures)	Sedation/BZD intoxication
			Donepezil	Loss of efficacy (dementia)	GI effects
			Escitalopram	Loss of efficacy (depression/anxiety)	GI effects
			Eszopiclone	Loss of efficacy (insomnia)	Sedation/confusion
			Flibanserin	Loss of efficacy (sexual desire)	Nausea/dizziness/sedation
			Flurazepam	Loss of efficacy (insomnia)	Sedation/BZD intoxication
			Galantamine	Loss of efficacy (dementia)	GI effects
			Guanfacine	Loss of efficacy (ADHD)	Sedation/dry mouth/dizziness
			Iloperidone	Loss of efficacy (psychosis)	Sedation/dizziness
			Levomilnacipran	Loss of efficacy (depression)	GI effects
			Loxapine	Loss of efficacy (psychosis)	EPS/sedation
			Lurasidone	Loss of efficacy (psychosis)	Sedation/akathisia
			Methadone	Opiate withdrawal	CNS and respiratory depression
			Mirtazapine	Loss of efficacy (depression/insomnia)	Somnolence
			Modafinil	Loss of efficacy (narcolepsy)	Insomnia/increased pulse
			Oral contraceptives	Loss of efficacy (pregnancy)	GI effects
			Pimavanserin	Loss of efficacy (psychosis)	Nausea/confusion
			Quetiapine	Loss of efficacy (psychosis)	Sedation/orthostasis
			Statins (not pravastatin)	Loss of efficacy (hyperlipidemia)	Rhabdomyolysis

CYP450 Family	Inducers	Inhibitors	Substrates ("Victim" Drugs)	Symptoms When Induced	Symptoms When Inhibited
3A4	Armodafinil Barbiturates Carbamazepine Modafinil Oxcarbazepine Phenytoin Rifampin St. John's wort (Topiramate)	Clarithromycin Fluconazole Fluvoxamine Grapefruit juice Ketoconazole Protease inhibitors	Sildenafil	Loss of efficacy (sexual dysfunction)	Headache/flushing/prolonged erection
			Suvorexant	Loss of efficacy (insomnia)	Sedation/confusion
			Tadalafil	Loss of efficacy (sexual dysfunction)	Headache/flushing/prolonged erection
			Tasimelteon	Loss of efficacy (insomnia)	Sedation
			Tiagabine	Loss of efficacy (seizures)	Dizziness/somnolence/difficulty concentrating
			Trazodone	Loss of efficacy (insomnia)	Sedation/orthostasis
			Triazolam	Loss of efficacy (insomnia/anxiety/seizures)	Sedation/BZD intoxication
			Tricyclics	Loss of efficacy (depression/anxiety)	Seizures/arrhythmia/anticholinergic
			Vardenafil	Loss of efficacy (sexual dysfunction)	Headache/flushing/prolonged erection
			Vilazodone	Loss of efficacy (depression/anxiety)	GI effects
			Zaleplon	Loss of efficacy (insomnia)	Sedation/confusion
			Ziprasidone	Loss of efficacy (psychosis)	Sedation/akathisia
			Zolpidem	Loss of efficacy (insomnia)	Sedation/confusion

( ) indicates less potent inhibitory effect, therefore generally less of a risk except at higher doses

APPENDIX B: PSYCHIATRIC MEDICATIONS IN PREGNANCY AND LACTATION

Determining the risk of medications in pregnancy used to be a simple matter of looking up a drug's pregnancy categorization in the PDR. This went from category "A", which is the lowest risk, to "X", which means the drug is contraindicated in pregnancy. But this ABCDX system provided very little practical or clinically useful information. In 2014, the FDA came up with a new system of labeling, which requires descriptive subsections on different aspects of pregnancy and lactation, and omits the letter categories—though you'll still see the old system in use for drugs approved before 2015.

Pregnancy presents a unique problem to the psychiatrist. Contrary to what many may think or assume, pregnancy does not protect a woman from an acute episode, a recurrence, or an exacerbation of psychiatric illness. Withholding medications during pregnancy can *sometimes* be an appropriate option, but this is generally not recommended. And since all psychotropic medications cross the placenta to at least *some* degree, their potential effects on the fetus, on labor and delivery, and on the neonate must be considered and balanced with the risk of *not* treating the mother with medication (see our July/August 2016 double issue of *TCPR* for an overview). A similar risk-benefit assessment must be considered in the case of a mother who wishes to breastfeed her child, as psychotropic medications are excreted into breast milk to varying degrees.

One of us (TP) is a pharmacist specializing in psychopharmacology, and commonly consulted by psychiatrists to provide updated information on the safety of medications in pregnancy and breastfeeding. It is a difficult task, because the quantity and quality of data vary greatly. The accompanying table was developed by pulling together a variety of sources, including isolated case reports, case series, birth registries, retrospective surveys, prospective comparative cohort studies, case control studies, and meta-analyses. Making judgments about which medication to use—or not use—in a pregnant or lactating woman is a delicate balancing act, involving an assessment of the severity of the underlying illness versus the uncertainties inherent in prescribing medications when the available data are limited.

In reading the table, keep the following in mind: In the general US population, the baseline rate of major malformations is between 1% and 4%, depending on the population studied and the definitions of "malformations" used. If treatment is necessary, monotherapy with the lowest *effective* dose and for the shortest duration is prudent. Safety data are generally more robust with older agents, and for that reason older agents—with a few key exceptions—are more preferable than newer drugs with less established safety profiles.

Almost all drugs enter breast milk. The exposure to the infant is described as a percentage of the maternal dose—that is, how much of the weight-adjusted maternal dose is actually excreted into the breast milk. When less than 10% of a mother's dose of medication is excreted into the breast milk, it is generally considered compatible with breastfeeding (with some exceptions) since these low serum levels are unlikely to lead to adverse effects in the infant.

While the table summarizes the current knowledge about psychotropic medication in pregnancy and lactation, information in this area is constantly evolving. If you regularly treat women of childbearing age, we suggest that you keep up with new data, consult with experts, and use resources such as the Organization of Teratology Information Specialists at www.mothertobaby.org or 866-626-6847; Motherisk at www.motherisk.org; or the LactMed peer reviewed database of the National Library of Medicine, updated monthly at http://1.usa.gov/15eWNH. Another good resource is the MGH Center for Women's Mental Health at www.womensmentalhealth.org. And, if you don't mind paying a fee (or if you are a trainee and have free access), you can check out www.reprotox.org, an online database of summaries. Another source of information can be the drug labeling, which, as of 2015, is more detailed than in the past. These resources, along with our table, provide information based upon the available evidence (or lack thereof), but the ultimate clinical decision comes down to careful and individualized consideration between the physician and the patient and her family.

Additional References

- Besag FM. ADHD treatment and pregnancy. *Drug Saf* 2014;37(6):397–408.
- Chisolm MS et al. Management of psychotropic drugs during pregnancy. *BMJ* 2016;352:h5918.
- Khan SJ et al. Bipolar disorder in pregnancy and postpartum: Principles of management. *Curr Psychiatry Rep* 2016;18(2):13.
- McLafferty LP et al. Guidelines for the management of pregnant women with substance use disorders. *Psychosomatics* 2016;57(2):115–130.
- Muzik M et al. Use of antidepressants during pregnancy?: What to consider when weighing treatment with antidepressants against untreated depression. *Matern Child Health J* 2016;20(11):2268–2279.

- Ornoy A et al. Antidepressant, antipsychotics, and mood stabilizers in pregnancy: What do we know and how should we treat pregnant women with depression? *Birth Defects Res* 2017:109(12):933–956.
- Oyebode F et al. Psychotropics in pregnancy: Safety and other considerations. *Pharmacol Ther* 2012;135(1):71–77.
- Payne JL. Psychopharmacology in pregnancy and breastfeeding. *Psychiatr Clin North Am* 2017;40(2):217–238.
- Rowe H et al. Maternal medication, drug use, and breastfeeding. *Child Adolesc Psychiatr Clin N Am* 2015;24(1):1–20.
- Sachs HC et al. The transfer of drugs and therapeutics into human breast milk: An update on selected topics. *Pediatrics* 2013;132(3):e796–e809.
- Vigod S et al. Depression in pregnancy. *BMJ* 2016;352:i547.

APPENDIX B TABLE: Psychiatric Medications in Pregnancy and Lactation

Medication	Pregnancy	Breastfeeding	Recommendations
Anxiolytics/hypnotics			
Benzodiazepines (various agents)	Possible increased incidence of cleft lip or palate (with first trimester exposure); floppy infant syndrome (with exposure just before delivery); neonatal withdrawal syndrome; lower Apgar scores	Excretion varies with different benzodiazepines, but it is always less than 10%. Excessive sedation in infant, lethargy with consequent feeding difficulty and weight loss reported.	Try to avoid use in first trimester and late in pregnancy (although intermittent use less likely to induce withdrawal symptoms in neonate). Lorazepam (Ativan) may be best in class to use due to lack of active metabolites and relatively shorter half-life. Monitor sedation in breastfed infants; use of shorter-acting agents preferred.
Buspirone (BuSpar)	Fewer data; difficult to determine risks	Low to undetectable infant levels reported	Due to lack of data, other agents with larger safety database should be considered first
Diphenhydramine (Benadryl)	Fairly consistent data show lack of associated malformations	Larger doses or more prolonged use may cause adverse effects in the infant	Considered to be the safest hypnotic in pregnancy and breastfeeding
Non-benzodiazepines: Eszopiclone (Lunesta) Zaleplon (Sonata) Zolpidem (Ambien)	Fewer data show no increased risk of malformations	Relatively low levels in breast milk. Most data are with zolpidem. Zolpidem is relatively hydrophilic and excreted rapidly; therefore, may be favored.	Reserve for second-line use due to paucity of data. If unavoidable, use zolpidem at lowest dose possible.
Suvorexant (Belsomra)	No data	No data	Best to use other agents with data and longer record of experience
Trazodone	Fewer data show no increased risk of malformations	<1% excretion; not expected to cause adverse effects in breastfed infants	Probably safe
Mood stabilizers			
Carbamazepine (Tegretol)	Rate of major malformation reported to be 2.2%–7.9%. Neural tube defects (0.5%–1%), craniofacial defects, cardiovascular malformations, and hypospadias reported.	Relatively high levels in breast milk but with few adverse effects reported. Sedation, poor sucking, withdrawal reactions, and 3 cases of hepatic dysfunction have been reported.	Avoid if possible. High-dose (4 mg) folic acid supplementation recommended.
Lamotrigine (Lamictal)	Rate of major malformations reported to be 1%–5.6%. Increased risk of oral clefts (0.4%).	Based on limited data, thought to be safe; however, infant exposure can be high and can vary widely (reports of 18%–60% of maternal concentrations); monitor infant. Relatively high infant exposure (22.7%); avoid or exercise caution.	Considered to be the safest of the anticonvulsants in pregnancy, though good safety data is sparse
Lithium (Eskalith, Lithobid)	Rate of major malformations reported to be 4%–12%. Increased risk of cardiovascular malformation, Ebstein's anomaly; risk is lower than previously thought (0.05%–0.1%). Increased maternal risk of diabetes, polyhydramnios, thyroid dysfunction during pregnancy.	30%–50% excretion; not recommended due to high risk of toxicity	Avoid, particularly in first trimester. Check serum levels and thyroid function frequently during pregnancy. Changes in metabolism and total body water necessitate frequent dose adjustment, particularly in third trimester. Avoid in breastfeeding if possible.
Oxcarbazepine (Trileptal)	Unlike carbamazepine, there is no epoxide metabolite formed, so oxcarbazepine may be less teratogenic; a Danish study showed no increased risk of major malformation. However, data with oxacarbazepine are limited.	Limited information suggests oxcarbazepine would not be expected to cause adverse effects in breastfed infants, especially if the infant is older than 2 months. Monitor infant for drowsiness, adequate weight gain, and developmental milestones, especially in younger, exclusively breastfed infants and when using combinations of anticonvulsants.	Use caution until more data available

Medication	Pregnancy	Breastfeeding	Recommendations
Valproate (Depakote)	Most teratogenic of all mood stabilizers, with a 6.2%–20.3% rate of congenital malformations, with neural tube defects most prominent. Teratogenic effects are dose-related with greatest risk at doses >1000 mg per day.	Relatively low excretion (0.68%); considered compatible with breastfeeding	Best to avoid in pregnancy unless absolutely required. High-dose (4 mg) folic acid supplementation recommended.
Antipsychotics			
Atypicals	Fewer data available, most showing no increased risk of malformations. Maternal hyperglycemia, impaired glucose tolerance, and weight gain may lead to maternal complications. Large-for-gestational-age infants reported. Floppy infant syndrome reported in clozapine exposure; monitor neutrophils in neonate for 6 months.	Excretion low, usually <3%, with exception of clozapine (Clozaril), which is seen in relatively high concentrations in breast milk	Overall, relatively safe in pregnancy; not treating serious mental illness in pregnancy poses greater risk. Most data with risperidone, olanzapine, quetiapine. Avoid clozapine in breastfeeding if possible.
Conventionals	No increased risk of malformations seen with high-potency agents. Small increased risk with low-potency agents such as chlorpromazine (Thorazine). Transient extrapyramidal side effects; sedation; withdrawal symptoms in neonates.	Relatively low excretion reported although little data available. Sedation and parkinsonism effects possible in breastfed infants.	Haloperidol (Haldol), fluphenazine (Prolixin) favored during pregnancy because of long history of safe use and fewer hypotensive, anticholinergic, and antihistaminergic effects. Limited data in breastfeeding; relatively safe.
Antidepressants			
Bupropion (Wellbutrin)	No increased risk of malformation shown thus far	<1% excretion with no adverse outcomes reported	Well characterized and considered reasonable option. May also help with smoking cessation during pregnancy.
Duloxetine (Cymbalta)	Little data	No published data, though exposure is low	Other agents with more data favored
Levomilnacipran (Fetzima)	No data	No published data	Other agents with more data favored
Mirtazapine (Remeron)	Sparse data, but one small study suggests no increased rate of major malformation	Low excretion; compatible with breastfeeding	May be useful also for pregnancy-associated emesis, insomnia
SSRIs	Controversial data regarding cardiovascular malformation with first trimester paroxetine (Paxil) exposure. Larger and more recent studies show no overall increased risk for malformations with SSRIs. Conflicting reports with some showing decreased gestational age, low birth weight, poor neonatal adaptation, low Apgar scores (some of which could be due to underlying depression or anxiety). Conflicting reports regarding SSRI use in later pregnancy and persistent pulmonary hypertension (PPHN). Neonatal toxicity reported as transient jitteriness, tremulousness, and tachypnea. No problems detected in behavioral or cognitive development—greatest data with fluoxetine (Prozac).	Relatively low excretion, varies by agent: Fluoxetine: 3%–9% Paroxetine: <4% Sertraline (Zoloft): <2% Citalopram (Celexa): 5%–10% Fluvoxamine (Luvox): <2%	Best studied and most used class of psychotropics in pregnancy. Relatively safe in pregnancy; avoid paroxetine if possible. Sertraline results in lowest fetal drug exposure and lowest (undetectable) levels in breastfed infants; may be considered favored SSRI. Paroxetine use most controversial. Fluoxetine less favored for breastfeeding due to long half-life and active metabolite; disturbed sleep, colic, irritability, poor feeding reported.
Tricyclics	Relatively large database; recent meta-analysis of 300,000 live births revealed no increased risk of malformations. Neonatal anticholinergic effects. Transient neonatal withdrawal symptoms reported.	<1%–5% excretion; appear relatively safe during breastfeeding, with possible exception of doxepin	Well characterized and considered reasonable options. Desipramine (Norpramin), nortriptyline (Pamelor) preferred due to lower anticholinergic and orthostatic hypotension risks. Monitor baby for sedation in breastfeeding.

Medication	Pregnancy	Breastfeeding	Recommendations
Venlafaxine/ desvenlafaxine (Pristiq)	Earlier data regarding major malformations reassuring, but one more recent study suggested a possible association with birth defects; additional studies needed. Increased maternal blood pressure may be a concern during pregnancy, particularly at higher doses.	2%–9.2% excretion; no adverse outcomes reported	Other agents with more data favored
Vilazodone (Viibryd)	No data	No published data	Other agents with more data favored
Vortioxetine (Trintellix)	No data	No published data	Other agents with more data favored
Stimulants			
Amphetamines and methylphenidate	No apparent congenital malformations; may constrict blood flow to placenta, which reduces oxygen flow to developing fetus. May cause premature delivery, small for gestational age and low-birth-weight babies; however, data inconclusive. Neonatal withdrawal possible.	0.2% excreted into breast milk; adverse effects usually not observed	Caution in pregnancy due to possibility of vasoconstriction and ability to disrupt blood flow to the fetus

APPENDIX C TABLE: SCHEDULES OF CONTROLLED SUBSTANCES

In 1970, under the Controlled Substance Act, the FDA created classification schedules that organize drugs into groups based on their risk of abuse or harm. There are 5 classifications of controlled substances (Schedule I, II, III, IV, and V), and drugs with the highest risk to benefit ratio are considered Schedule I drugs. Most drugs used in psychiatry are not scheduled at all (antidepressants, antipsychotics, etc.). Some of us get confused about whether the most restricted drugs are Schedule I or V. Here's a mnemonic: The number 1 looks like a needle, and a needle is used to inject heroin—which is the prototypical Schedule I drug.

Prescription drug monitoring programs (PDMPs) are searchable databases that can help prescribers identify potential abuse or diversion of controlled substances. If you prescribe controlled substances like benzodiazepines and stimulants, it's a good idea to learn about your state's PDMP laws, consider your search results in the context of all available information, and watch for regulatory changes over the next few years. To find your state's program, check with the PDMP Training and Technical Assistance Center (http://www.pdmpassist.org/content/state-pdmp-websites).

Schedule	Description	Prescribing Implications	Some Examples
I	No accepted medical use, high potential for abuse, illegal to possess or use	Can't be prescribed at all (with the exception of medical marijuana in some states)	Heroin, LSD, ecstasy, and others Marijuana (though legalized in some states, it is still illegal at the federal level)
II	High potential for abuse, but legal for medical use	Can be prescribed only 1 month at a time, cannot be refilled, cannot be called in, and patient must give pharmacy a paper script (unless you use an e-prescribing program that is certified by DEA to allow prescribing of controlled substances)	All psychostimulants, such as amphetamine and methylphenidate Opiates that are especially potent, such as oxycodone, fentanyl, and others Vicodin (hydrocodone and acetaminophen) was recently reclassified from Schedule III to Schedule II
III	Lower potential for abuse than Schedule I or II, but still pretty abusable	Can be refilled up to 5 times (no more than 6 months), can be called in	Suboxone (buprenorphine/naloxone) Ketamine Xyrem (sodium oxybate) Anabolic steroids Barbiturates Dronabinol (Marinol)
IV	Lower potential for abuse than Schedule III	Can be refilled up to 5 times (no more than 6 months), can be called in	All benzodiazepines (eg, clonazepam, lorazepam, etc.) Various hypnotics, such as zolpidem, zaleplon, and suvorexant (Belsomra) Wake-promoting agents, like modafinil and armodafinil Tramadol (Ultram) Carisoprodol (Soma) Lorcaserin (Belviq), an anti-obesity drug
V	Lowest potential for abuse	Can be refilled as many times as prescriber chooses (eg, for 1 year or more), can be called in	Pregabalin (Lyrica) Cough preparations with small amounts of codeine, such as Robitussin AC Antidiarrheal Lomotil (diphenoxylate/atropine)

An updated and more complete list of the schedules is published annually in Title 21 *Code of Federal Regulations* and can be found here: www.deadiversion.usdoj.gov/21cfr/cfr/2108cfrt.htm

APPENDIX D TABLE: LAB MONITORING FOR PSYCHIATRIC MEDICATIONS

This is a short and sweet table listing the medications that most psychiatrists would agree require lab monitoring. Our recommendations are quite abbreviated, and we haven't spelled out whether you should order labs before or after starting the medications, nor how you should do follow-up monitoring. There's just too much variation in practice for us to give authoritative detailed guidelines. These medications are mainly here to jog your memory, so you don't forget to at least consider what type of monitoring to do.

Medications	Recommended Laboratory Tests
Acamprosate	BUN/creatinine if renal impairment is suspected
Amantadine	BUN/creatinine if renal impairment is suspected
Antipsychotics—second generation, primarily clozapine, olanzapine, quetiapine, paliperidone, risperidone[1]	Fasting glucose and lipids
Atomoxetine	LFTs
Carbamazepine	CBZ level, complete blood count (CBC), sodium, LFTs, pregnancy test, HLA-B*1502 in Asians[2]
Chlorpromazine	ECG if cardiac disease
Citalopram	ECG if cardiac disease, dose $\geq$40 mg/day
Clozapine	Fasting glucose and lipids, CBC
Desvenlafaxine	Periodic BP
Deutetrabenazine	ECG if cardiac disease
Disulfiram	LFTs if liver disease is suspected
Duloxetine	LFTs if liver disease is suspected[3]
Gabapentin	BUN/creatinine if renal impairment is suspected
Levomilnacipran	Periodic BP/pulse rate
Lithium	Li level, TSH, BUN/creatinine[4], pregnancy test, ECG if cardiac disease
Methadone	ECG if cardiac disease
Mirtazapine	Lipids
Naltrexone	LFTs if liver disease is suspected
Oxcarbazepine	Sodium, HLA-B*1502 in Asians[5]
Paliperidone	Prolactin if symptoms, fasting glucose and lipids
Pregabalin	BUN/creatinine if renal impairment is suspected
Risperidone	Prolactin if symptoms, fasting glucose and lipids
SSRIs	Sodium in elderly if fatigue, dizziness, confusion
Stimulants	ECG if cardiac disease
Thioridazine	ECG if cardiac disease
Topiramate	Bicarbonate
Tricyclic antidepressants	ECG if cardiac disease
Valbenazine	ECG if cardiac disease
Valproic acid	VPA level, LFTs, CBC for platelets, pregnancy test, ammonia if confusion
Venlafaxine	Periodic BP
Ziprasidone	ECG if cardiac disease

[1] Some guidelines recommend monitoring glucose and lipids with all SGAs.

[2] HLA-B*1502 is a gene that increases the risk of developing toxic epidermal necrolysis (TEN) and Stevens-Johnson syndrome (SJS) in response to taking carbamazepine. Asians, especially the Han Chinese, are much more likely to have the gene than other populations.

[3] Duloxetine should not be prescribed in patients with significant alcohol use or evidence of chronic liver disease as it can lead to hepatic failure in rare cases (Cymbalta prescribing information). While the manufacturer does not recommend baseline LFTs for all patients, some clinicians do so anyway to be extra cautious.

[4] The serum creatinine is used to compute the estimated glomerular filtration rate (eGFR), a more precise measure of kidney functioning. Increasingly, laboratory test results include the estimated GFR. You can calculate it yourself using an online calculator at https://www.niddk.nih.gov/health-information/communication-programs/nkdep/laboratory-evaluation/glomerular-filtration-rate-calculators.

[5] HLA-B*1502 is a gene that increases the risk of developing toxic epidermal necrolysis (TEN) and Stevens-Johnson syndrome (SJS) in response to taking carbamazepine. Asians, especially the Han Chinese, are much more likely to have the gene than other populations.

APPENDIX E: PHARMACOGENETIC TESTING

The Basics

Variations in patients' genetic profiles can affect how they respond to medications. While the actual clinical importance of this phenomenon is not yet clear, it's likely that genetic variations in pharmacokinetic genes have some effect on serum levels of medications in many patients. Based on these CYP450 polymorphisms, individuals are categorized in different ways with respect to specific enzymes:

Extensive metabolizers: Otherwise known as "normal" metabolizers, these people have normally active CYP450 genes on both chromosomes, meaning that they see an average level of drug in the body.

Intermediate metabolizers: These people metabolize drugs a bit more slowly than extensive metabolizers, but not dramatically so.

Poor metabolizers: These people carry inactive or partially active CYP450 genes, and therefore metabolize drugs significantly more slowly than extensive metabolizers. This may result in more side effects since serum drug levels are higher.

Ultrarapid metabolizers: With extra copies of certain genes, these people metabolize drugs more quickly than extensive metabolizers, sometimes requiring unusually high doses of medications to achieve a therapeutic level.

There are also genetic variations in pharmacodynamic genes that might increase or decrease the efficacy of drugs, but the evidence for this effect is less robust than for pharmacokinetic effects.

Pharmacogenetic Testing in Clinical Practice

The science of pharmacogenetic testing is complex, which makes it hard for us mere mortals to evaluate the claims of the many commercial test kits flooding the market.

In March 2017, *TCPR* explored this topic and focused on three tests: Genesight, Genecept, and CNSDose. We concluded that the evidence was not yet robust enough to recommend any of these tests. However, we did review information from FDA drug labels and created a table listing FDA recommendations for pharmacogenetic testing relevant to specific psychotropic drugs.

Many of the recommendations are to lower starting doses in patients who are poor metabolizers. For example, in aripiprazole's label, you'll read: "Dosing recommendation in patients who are classified as CYP450 2D6 poor metabolizers (PM): The aripiprazole dose in PM patients should initially be reduced to one-half (50%) of the usual dose and then adjusted to achieve a favorable clinical response."

While the FDA does not specifically ask you to order genetic testing, you will not know whether your patient is a poor metabolizer unless someone has ordered it. Therefore, a case could be made for selectively ordering CYP450 testing to ensure you dose drugs in accordance with FDA labeling. Whether you do this is a judgment call; most of us are content to skip the genetic testing, and instead choose to start most medications at a low dose and titrate up gradually in order to prevent side effects.

APPENDIX E TABLE: FDA Label Information Relevant to Pharmacogenetic Testing for Psychiatric Drugs

Medication	FDA Recommendations	Clinical Rationale
Aripiprazole Atomoxetine Brexpiprazole Iloperidone Perphenazine Vortioxetine	Reduce dose in CYP2D6 PMs.[1]	Usual starting dose is too high in PMs, so start lower and increase gradually.
Amitriptyline Clomipramine Clozapine Desipramine Doxepin Imipramine Nortriptyline Protriptyline Trimipramine	Monitor levels in CYP2D6 PMs.	These medications, most of which are tricyclic antidepressants, can cause life-threatening side effects if levels are too high. Consider monitoring serum levels in PMs.
Citalopram	Maximum recommended daily dose of 20 mg (rather than 40 mg) for CYP2C19 PMs.	Risk of QT prolongation and cardiac arrhythmia.
Thioridazine	Contraindicated in CYP2D6 PMs, due to risk of QT prolongation.	Risk of QT prolongation and cardiac arrhythmia.
Pimozide	In CYP2D6 PMs, dose should not exceed 4 mg/day in adults.	Risk of QT prolongation and cardiac arrhythmia.
Carbamazepine Oxcarbazepine	Avoid or use cautiously in individuals with the HLA-B*1502 allele (applicable to Asians).	Risk of serious rashes such as Stevens-Johnson syndrome.

[1]PM = poor metabolizer

Source: http://www.fda.gov/Drugs/ScienceResearch/ResearchAreas/Pharmacogenetics/ucm083378.htm

Index

Note: Trade names are capitalized, bolded page numbers are for fact sheets, and non-bolded page numbers are for quick scan tables.